PRAISE FOR *HEAL AND GROW*

"Tremendous gratitude for *Heal and Grow*! Compassionate, humble, and wise, Jones shares his brave journey and caring heart to reveal epiphanies for us all to learn from."
—Dana Marie Lupton, cofounder of Moving in the Spirit

"If you're looking for the clarity, inspiration, and guidance you need to become a better version of yourself, read this book! Jones shares stories that let you know that you're not alone in any struggle you may be facing. . . . He offers solid, actionable advice that will guide you through challenges on your own and help you see when you might need additional support on your healing journey. This book feels like an honest, kind, and supportive friend who only wants the best for you—to 'heal and grow.'"
—Jeanne Sparrow, speaker, consultant, TV/radio personality

"*Heal and Grow* centers on something that I strive for every day—inner peace. I was moved when Jones referenced how we cannot ignore spirituality when searching for it. I am excited to be able to share how *Heal and Grow* can and will help me to grow—as well as you."
—Elroy Smith, director of urban content, Cox Media Group

"Jones, in his new book *Heal and Grow*, shares his process of becoming a psychotherapist and answers his question, 'Why did I decide to become a psychotherapist anyway?' He offers helpful lessons learned through his twenty years of service to others. The book is uplifting and serves as a guide to preventing burnout. It is a book that I found healing and inspiring."

—Trudy Post Sprunk, LMFT&S, LPC, CPCS,
SEP, EMDR Certified, RPT&S

HEAL AND GROW

HEAL AND GROW

Lessons Learned on My Journey as a Mental Health Professional

F. FRANCIS JONES

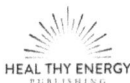

HEAL THY ENERGY
PUBLISHING

Published by Heal Thy Energy Publishing, Clarkston, Georgia
www.ffrancisjones.com

GIRL FRIDAY
PRODUCTIONS˚

Edited and designed by Girl Friday Productions
www.girlfridayproductions.com

Cover design by Rachael Brandenburg
Cover photo by F. Francis Jones
Project management: Sara Spees Addicott
Editorial production: Abi Pollokoff

ISBN (paperback): 979-8-9895634-0-1
ISBN (ebook): 979-8-9895634-1-8

Library of Congress Control Number: 2024901344

First edition

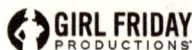

To Carla Edmonson, my cousin and, more importantly, my friend. At the age of only twenty-six, you were taken away from us far too soon. You will forever be missed, cherished, and loved.

To the people whose lives have been changed forever due to a loved one being taken away at the hands of someone who was unable, or unwilling, to get the emotional and mental health support they so desperately needed.

To the many people who have ended their lives due to being overwhelmed by their thoughts, feelings, pain, or life's challenges; as well as those they've left behind.

And to anyone who has been significantly impacted or challenged trying to support loved ones struggling with emotional or mental health issues.

CONTENTS

PREFACE

The world is changed by your example, not by your opinion.

—Paulo Coelho

Let me take you back to the summer of 2001. I was working as an associate producer for the show *Divorce Court* and feeling extremely stressed out. You see, a part of my job was to find couples willing to come on the program and create "good television" by sharing their conflicts and issues. Unfortunately, I was feeling significant pressure to book multiple eligible couples before the next taping date. In reality, I think the bigger issue wasn't necessarily about me running out of time; instead, the issue was about me doing something out of alignment with who I was—or who I wanted to be. I wanted my work to benefit others in a positive way. I also wanted to help people overcome their personal issues and challenges so they could lead happier lives. Then came the day when I gained a new sense of clarity.

I was talking to a wife who was a potential candidate for an upcoming episode. Soon, however, it became apparent that she and her estranged husband would likely not be suitable for our show (for a variety of reasons). After talking to this stressed-out and lonely woman for at least an hour, I was struck by a comment she made as our phone call came to a close. Despite being informed that she would not be selected for the program, she genuinely thanked me for simply being willing to listen. She felt truly appreciative of the fact that someone took the time to be there for her. Her words affected me deeply and gave me a new goal to help me make it through my challenging job.

From that day forward, my objective changed. No longer would I scour the nation for argumentative and brokenhearted couples to feature on our program. Instead, I made it my secret mission to do whatever I could to provide hope and even be a blessing by being present for couples in pain. I wanted to provide the service of compassion, or at least strive to. I no longer stressed about whether or not I had been able to book my share of couples for future episodes. I simply trusted that the universe and my belief in a Creator (divine intelligence) would allow me to successfully do my job in booking couples. In the meantime, I found a new motivation for getting up and going to work every day, which was something I had not experienced since I started working there. I was going to commit to being of service to others.

Unfortunately, about a month later, the tragic events of 9/11 took place. The production of *Divorce Court*, like so many other things, was brought to a screeching halt. People spent hour after hour watching news reports, trying to find answers to the devastation. The nation was in shock, confused, saddened—even angry. As the reality surrounding the events sunk in, people attempted to deal with the shock and disbelief. For those of us old enough to remember, planes were not allowed to fly for a period of time. And even when they were able to take to the skies again, many people were reluctant or outright refused to board a flight. Since *Divorce Court* flew many of our couples and guests to Southern California for taping, it became extremely difficult to convince some people to get on an airplane even though a variety of new security measures were now in place.

Ultimately, the show's entire production stopped, and by December approximately half of the staff was released. Despite no longer being employed, I realized that I was now presented with an opportunity to discover the career I truly wanted. The thing that would give me purpose and fulfillment. The job that I hoped would bring me joy by being able to serve others. Eventually, I decided that since it felt so rewarding listening to and supporting potential guests for the show, why not become a counselor? This, of course, required me to get a master's degree, which began a journey that included finding internships, studying for exams, writing papers, and eventually taking a licensing exam. Despite the long road I was about to travel, this new career direction felt like the right decision for me.

INTRODUCTION

*I used to worry too much about whether or
not I was supported, and not enough about
whether or not I was actively supporting others.*

—Marianne Williamson

Everyone's life journey has a starting point. Before I share
some of the many insights I've learned as a licensed mental
health professional, I thought it would be a good idea to let
you know a little bit about me, including my past and how I
became a therapist in the first place.

I was born in and grew up on the South Side of Chicago.
Until I was about nine years old, I was raised in a house with
my mother, father, and older sister. I don't recall a whole lot,
but I do remember the main vibe: it was *not* an idyllic upbringing resembling a Norman Rockwell painting. My father displayed one of two modes: either he was emotionally distant,
or he was controlling and abusive. This was especially true if
he had been drinking, which seemed to be, to my young eyes,
quite often. Apparently, my dad was very good with machinery
and figuring things out, which is why he worked as a station-
ary engineer. My mother, meanwhile, despite never finishing
elementary school, did the best she could with trying to bring
in additional money by working as a short-order cook. Neither

parent spent a significant amount of one-on-one time with me, which is why I often considered one our German shepherds my best friend. My sister, who is seven years older than me, did interact with me on some occasions, but she was frequently not home because my father would literally kick her out of the house and force her to live with other people or family members when he was in one of his angry or drunken states. I'm sure this made it very difficult for her to live anything close to a normal adolescent life. My father (who was not her biological parent) often took out a lot of his anger, abusive tendencies, and controlling ways on my sister and mom. Eventually, our mother was able to escape with my sister and me to another part of the city where, for several years, we lived in fear while hoping and praying he would never find us. I can't speak for my mother and sister, but I always thought that if he ever found us, we would be either physically punished or forced to go back and live with him.

I've often wondered if growing up in this environment contributed to my wanting to save or rescue others from difficult situations. I have come to believe that we all have experiences and conditions from our past that we're trying to heal from. I've always sought to feel valued, special, and appreciated. To be quite honest, I still desire some degree of validation from time to time—like most people, I presume.

By the time I got to high school (shout-out to South Shore High School), I was pretty much a shy and introverted kid, especially if the environment and other kids were new to me. I had friends in the neighborhood, and one eventually became my best friend. Interacting and hanging out with the kids in my neighborhood usually meant playing a variety of games, often outside. We'd play sports and board games, read Marvel comics, race slot cars, and engage in thrilling rounds of hide-and-seek. That is, if I was fortunate enough for my mom to allow me to stay out despite the streetlights being on.

In high school, I found that it took some time before I was able to develop close relationships. Academically, I got average grades despite being in the honors program. Before you jump to any conclusions that I was some sort of supersmart student, I assure you that was not the case. It's just that the public school I attended was considered, at best, to be an average to below-average place to get an education. I just so happened to have high reading scores from consuming so many comic books as a kid, so I typically did well on standardized tests. To be quite frank, I feel like I struggled throughout high school—academically and socially. And having a girlfriend was practically impossible for me. I didn't have my first official girlfriend until my senior year.

However, something very important took place in high school that I believe placed me on this journey of being a mental health professional. Somehow, I became the person whom many of my peers brought their problems to. If you're reading this book, you may have also experienced something similar. And this is especially true if you're a therapist or have ever thought about becoming one. The types of problems my fellow teens brought to me were usually boyfriend-girlfriend relationship issues, some dispute between two friends, or challenges they were experiencing within their home. Whatever the reason or situation was, I liked listening and trying to help them find solutions. I particularly enjoyed it when those bringing their problems to me were girls. Deep down, I felt that if I could be there for them, supporting them with their issues, then somehow it would endear me to them. Well, it worked— sort of. But not in the way I had hoped. The girls typically were very fond of me and appreciated me being there for them, but going forward they only saw me as a good friend. I was often told, "You're like a brother to me." Nothing like going through high school and being stuck in the friend zone with the majority of girls I knew.

HIGHER LEARNING

Once I graduated from high school, I soon found myself in college majoring in communications at Southern Illinois University at Carbondale, with a focus on radio and television. During the second semester of my freshman year, I took one psychology course. I found it fascinating and would often read topics not discussed in the lectures from throughout the textbook. However, despite how much I enjoyed this class, I ended up with a D. I then told myself, "Well, I guess I clearly don't have what it takes to become a therapist." This reaffirmed for me that a career in radio and television was the path I should take.

I transferred to Columbia College in Chicago, where I completed my last two years of college and obtained my bachelor's degree. While there, I was able to get an internship at the top R&B radio station in Chicago, WGCI. Upon graduation, they immediately hired me as a full-time employee. I worked in various departments (from marketing and promotions to production) and eventually became an on-air personality going by the name Frankie J. I truly enjoyed working in radio—at least most of the time. However, I often felt a strong desire to do more. Somehow, I wanted to make a bigger difference. In my midtwenties there were so many times I found myself praying and asking God to help me become a person who changes people's lives for the better.

After working in radio for about seven years, I soon found myself transitioning to the world of television. This involved me relocating to Southern California and working on a variety of shows. Ultimately, I had enough of doing that as well, and after leaving *Divorce Court* (my final television show), I realized that going back to college, getting my master's degree, and becoming a licensed mental health professional was how I wanted to serve others. Once I had this realization, I shared it with my closest friends. None of them were surprised to hear about my decision. As a matter of fact, one of my friends even questioned why it took so long for me to get to this point, especially since I was always reading self-help books and trying to be a supportive, pretend therapist for many of my friends anyway.

MY PROFESSIONAL JOURNEY BEGINS

Going to graduate school in Southern California, studying for tests, and keeping up with various homework assignments while having a full-time job and two internships was extremely challenging for me. I consider it to be one of the most difficult periods of my life. I was often, if not always, tired, drained, and forced to put the rest of my life on hold.

Fortunately, this was only two years of my life, and I would eventually graduate and begin my journey in earnest as a therapist. I ended up working and gaining experience in a variety of settings that included treating teens in group homes and working at a day-treatment center (where young children with severe emotional or mental issues came every day after school).

After living in the Los Angeles area for seven years, I decided I'd had enough of the traffic and of being so far away from my friends and family in Chicago. To be honest, I was also frustrated with the unending romantic drought as I struggled to find a girlfriend or even anything that resembled a close relationship. I would occasionally get a first date with someone, but for some reason second dates never seemed to happen. This left me feeling unfulfilled and lonely. I eventually decided to relocate to Atlanta for a few reasons: One, I knew it was beautiful, and I could experience the change of seasons without the harsh winters of Chicago. Two, I knew a few people who lived there. Three, it would ultimately make it much easier to visit my family and friends in the Windy City. In Georgia, I continued to gain experience as a therapist and eventually (after my second try) passed my marriage and family therapy licensing exam. My resume grew as I took advantage of my opportunities to work in new and challenging settings, which included in-home and school-based treatment for children, a residential facility, and two private practices.

Despite all the experience I was gaining, I wanted to do something in addition to being a licensed therapist. One night I woke up somewhere around two or three in the morning and found it difficult to fall back to sleep. I decided to pull out my Kindle and watch some random YouTube videos. On this particular night, I felt an urge to watch something motivational, which led me to view a lecture by a man I've admired for years, Dr. Dennis Kimbro.

Dr. Kimbro is a motivational speaker, bestselling author, and professor at Clark Atlanta University. I've read some of his books and heard him speak in person—on several occasions, he was the guest speaker on days I delivered sermons at a church I attended in Chicago.

As I listened to him speak in a lecture hall at Clark Atlanta University one day, a thought suddenly occurred to me: *I'd like to do what he's doing.* I would continue providing mental health services, but if I could become a college instructor, I could reach more people (in this case, college students) in the hopes of making a positive difference. Instead of just meeting individuals and families, perhaps I could become an adjunct college instructor, I thought. The next morning, I reached out to a former coworker who was working at a college in my area. As luck would have it, she informed me that her department currently had an opening. Without going through all of the details here, I was eventually hired and, to date, have spent more than five years teaching basic psychology at this community college.

Although there have been a few challenges here and there, it has been a wonderful experience overall. It is my hope that my students have been able to not only learn about the fundamentals of psychology but also learn to better understand people and, more importantly, better understand themselves.

WHY I DECIDED TO BECOME A THERAPIST

Being a therapist definitely has its challenging moments. If you work in the field of mental health, you know exactly what I mean. If you don't, just know that everyone has their own personal issues, history, drama, pain, and wounds that they are trying to overcome or work through. Despite these complexities, being a therapist has provided me with many benefits. It is not uncommon that when you're trying to support others to heal and grow, you're also healing and growing as well. I've learned that through serving so many different types of people (people from different nationalities, communities, genders, sexual orientations, and ages), I'm also gaining new insights. I truly strive to have a greater sense of appreciation for the things in my life, especially since I know what the lives of so many others look like. I've also gained a significant amount of experience learning about mindsets and how to zero in on specific or deeper problems, and I've improved my ability to identify possible solutions and effective interventions.

I remember one day, before I began my morning meditation, I found myself unexpectedly tearing up. It occurred to me why I was driven to be a mental health professional. First of all, I have always had a strong desire to connect with others. Unfortunately, throughout my life there were plenty of times when this strong desire went unmet. This is probably why I've created an additional family, or what one might refer to as a surrogate family. From high school to this very day, I have gained an aunt, an uncle, two sisters, and two nieces whom I'm not biologically related to. Despite this reality, they've become as important to me as blood relatives. I truly see them as my family, and I love them very much for the amazing impact they've had on my life. The reason I felt compelled to create a family of my own choosing was reflected in the family void I'd had, which I was finally coming to terms with, and the realization of my early loss made me utterly sad.

A second reason that drove me to become a counselor is what I refer to as the "superhero complex." Let me take a moment to define this. It might be something you've seen in others, or perhaps you might recognize this trait in yourself. I consider someone to have a superhero complex when they have a strong desire to support, save, or rescue others who are typically experiencing some sort of crisis. Oftentimes, the desire is so strong that the individual will do whatever they feel needs to be done to help, even if it means they become stressed or inconvenienced in the process. Now, this strong desire to self-sacrifice may sound like an amazing trait—something that could benefit our society if there were more people willing to put others first. However, many things come with a price, and being a superhero definitely does. Individuals who typically play this role tend to try to rescue often and end up becoming emotionally, mentally, or even physically burned out. We rarely, if ever, say no when people come to us in need. Yes, the superhero needs to develop boundaries, but that is something learned over time. Thankfully, I have made significant progress in this area.

As Pollyannaish as this may sound, I have always wanted to save the world, help people, and make this world a better place. As long as we're willing to try to help people heal, grow, and accomplish their goals, things can and will change for the positive. These changes are definitely possible if, in addition to evolving as individuals and humans, we can demonstrate more kindness, understanding, and love toward one another.

The final reason I became a therapist is I want to matter. Perhaps you do as well. To varying degrees, we all want to feel valued, appreciated, significant, and important. I don't know if any or all of these are selfish reasons for wanting to be a therapist and serve others, but I have to be honest and admit they're true for me.

Many years have passed since I decided to leave the world of radio and television and become a mental health professional. I have now been a licensed marriage and family therapist for more than twenty years. I have seen, heard, and experienced a variety of things all while trying to help people to heal and grow—or better yet, to "grow through" their perceived personal challenges.

THE REASONING BEHIND THIS BOOK

My life has been deeply enriched by being a part of other people's lives, so I decided to share some of the many insightful things I've learned while being of service to others as a mental health professional. There are several objectives I'm hoping to achieve with this book. First, I will detail portions of my sometimes challenging yet amazing journey as a licensed marriage and family therapist. Second, I hope that those who may have once been fearful of or reluctant to consider therapy become open to the possibility that getting treatment could be beneficial and lead to a turning point in overcoming or dealing with their personal challenges. Lastly, through these pages, I hope you are encouraged and inspired to find ways to overcome, heal from, and grow through your life experiences. Perhaps those seeking to one day become clinicians may also find this material useful. The bottom line is that this book is another way for me to assist people. Hopefully, it will stimulate some positive changes within our world. A world that increasingly needs more healing, more understanding, more caring, and more love than ever before.

I don't believe I could have written this book ten years ago, five years ago, or even one year ago. The idea had not occurred to me to even do so; I simply wasn't inspired or led by the spirit within me to create a book. However, like many people, I thought it sounded appealing to write one, but I never knew what to write about. That is, until I realized I had something to share.

Over the years, I've tried to help many people deal with difficult situations. As a result, I've learned plenty. My clients have provided inspiration, perspective, and insight into a variety of issues they were dealing with. I've always sought out information and material that would support me in my continued personal development and journey. This has included books, movies, TV shows, random sayings, conversations with friends, religious sermons, and even thoughts that come to me during my daily morning meditations (this happens quite frequently). I would then selectively share what I have learned with others, especially if there was something they could benefit from as well.

Now that you've learned about me, my past, and how I got here, let me briefly share a little bit about what to expect in the upcoming chapters. Throughout this book I'll be sharing what I've learned as a mental health therapist while dedicating my life to helping individuals, couples, and families. To be more specific, I'll disclose my observations about working with men in therapy and what anxiety and depression have looked like for many of my clients. I will share how I work with people and identify possible interventions that may promote healing and growth. I'll offer my thoughts regarding the importance of self-care, the challenges I've experienced in therapy, my hopes for the future, and other topics that I hope you will find interesting if not enlightening. From this point on, the remaining chapters do not have to be read in any specific order. Each chapter has its own focus, so read them in any order you see fit, or simply read the next section that is calling your attention.

You may find questions arising about your loved ones, your past, your personal experiences, and your individual life challenges. If this occurs, I encourage you to try to find the strength to look inside and be honest with yourself. I also suggest that you be vulnerable and open to seeking help from others if you need it or if it could be beneficial for you. Know that help does not have to come in the form of a therapist or mental health professional. We can also gain something from speaking with others, which could include teachers, ministers, open-minded family members, and friends. We all can benefit from having someone there to listen, provide support, assist with our struggles, and encourage our attempts to heal. However, and I can't stress this enough, if you are in any way struggling with emotional or mental health issues that are making it extremely difficult to make it through the day, please seek professional help.

If you or someone you know is feeling suicidal, I strongly encourage you to contact 911 or get to an emergency room as soon as possible. There is also the National Suicide and Crisis Lifeline, where a trained counselor is available twenty-four hours a day to assist anyone experiencing a severe mental health crisis. As of July 2022, this crisis line can be accessed by dialing 988.

This book contains my personal thoughts, experiences, observations, and journey—along with a few insightful quotes. For most of my life, I've tried to serve others while also continuing my own growth. It is not my intention to tell you how you should or shouldn't live your life. I'm also not here to tell fellow clinicians, coaches, parents, or those who are in a

position to provide support what they need to do. I am sharing and hoping you gain something positive from these pages.
In the words of one of my childhood heroes, martial artist
and actor Bruce Lee, when it comes to the information in this
book, "absorb what is useful." Please allow what is presented
here to assist you in considering new ideas and new actions
to take. May your refined actions create positive change or a
difference in how you interact with others and how you view
yourself. We should all strive to take care of ourselves while
also supporting the healing of others. If we are all able to do
this, then perhaps one day we'll have a world that is kinder and
demonstrates more unity.

CHAPTER 1

Lessons Learned About People and Therapy

Tensions often dramatically decrease once someone knows that he has space to be heard.

—Kelli Harding, MD, MPH

While I was pursuing my master's in psychology, my fellow classmates and I were strongly encouraged by our professors to be in therapy (if we weren't already doing so). They wanted us to experience what it felt like to be the one sitting on the couch—in other words, the client. The professors also felt it would be a good idea because we all have issues that we need to address. I really wasn't sure what I wanted to discuss in a therapy session, but I liked the fact that for every hour of therapy we took, we earned three practicum hours, and if I recall

correctly, we needed 150 hours in order to graduate. So anything that got me closer to that number, I was all for it.

I have no memory of how I went about finding a therapist. Was it through the internet, a magazine, my school, or a
recommendation? I simply can't recall. I do remember I was
living in Burbank, California, at the time and had a full-time
job in south Los Angeles. For some reason, I decided to see a
clinician who was in Beverly Hills. Now, if you're not familiar
with Southern California, let me just say that all three of these
locations are easily forty-five minutes to an hour away from
one another. Therefore dealing with LA traffic was unavoid-
able, no matter what time of the day it was. Ultimately, I spoke
to a licensed clinician on the phone and agreed to make an
appointment to see her in the morning before going to work.
I arrived at the therapist's office (a few minutes late!), and for
a large portion of the time, I couldn't stop thinking about the
hour-plus drive it took me to get through the morning commute. I was cordial and answered all of her questions as honestly as possible. However, in my head I was also trying to
determine how much time it would take me to cross town to
get to my job at Challengers Boys & Girls Club on time in the
area that used to be called South Central LA. The therapist
had a calming demeanor and was very nice overall. However,
when I explained to her that this probably wouldn't be a good
match due to the drive, she immediately (and repeatedly)
started suggesting that I was making these comments because deep down I had some inner problem (or problems) that
I was reluctant to deal with in therapy. No matter how hard
I tried to convince her that this was not the case, she continued trying to press the issue. Of course, I eventually left that
office, and when I did, I knew my first visit to see her was also
going to be my last.

Thankfully, I found another therapist whose office was
much closer to where I lived and who also turned out to be a

better fit. As a result, we were able to explore a lot of my personal challenges, including my lack of a romantic relationship, loneliness, and childhood without a father or father figure. This was when it became apparent to me that every clinician is not a fit for every person.

In this chapter I'll share what I've learned about providing treatment as a mental health clinician, including some of the reasons why people decide to go to therapy, the possible benefits, and the situations that clients have typically brought to my office. I'll also share various tools and interventions I have used in treatment.

THE NEED FOR THERAPY

Let me start by stating the obvious: life can be very challenging. Many of us go through periods where we struggle to deal with what's going on in our outer world, which then negatively impacts what's going on inside of us. Or perhaps it's the reverse, and we find ourselves wrestling with internal struggles (e.g., things from our past) that make it difficult to manage what's currently going on around us, such as a relationship or a job. These challenges can cause us to experience pain and discomfort, making it extremely difficult to deal with our day-to-day lives.

There are many people who, on the outside, always have a great attitude or a smile on their faces; what we don't see is the internal battle going on within them. This is why it's beneficial for all of us to learn to identify ways to deal with, better understand, and effectively manage our emotions and feelings—regardless of what has taken place in our lives, our communities, and the world. If we don't, our thoughts and situations can potentially become overwhelming and prevent us from experiencing the peace, joy, and happiness we all desire.

This is where the trained mental health clinician could play a beneficial role.

Ideally, there would be no need for people like me. In a perfect world, whatever the personal struggles you or I may be going through, we would have people we could turn to for help. Some of us are fortunate enough to have such individuals. However, for many of us, there are few people (if any) who are in our corner; are willing to listen objectively, without judgment and without criticism; and refrain from trying to tell us what they think we should or shouldn't do. It can also be challenging to share with others because we're embarrassed or feel ashamed of our situation or actions.

Going to therapy and having someone to talk to can potentially prevent what I refer to as "the pop." Allow me to explain. When working with children, I often try to share with them the benefits of being in therapy and coming to see someone like me. If they are struggling with emotions such as anger or depression, I share my "balloon metaphor." I calmly ask, "What happens when you put too much air into a balloon?" Of course, they say, "It pops!" Then I explain that when we hold certain emotions inside, it can cause us to one day pop as well. I tell them that although we may not pop like balloons, there are ways that people pop too. This may include being overcome by sadness, crying, becoming angry, breaking things, or maybe even hurting someone. Perhaps for some, the pop may lead to engaging in behaviors that are risky and potentially harmful (to them or to someone else).

I've also shared this metaphor with adults, and when I do, the examples I include are excessive drinking, drug use, promiscuity, reckless shopping or overspending, or other behaviors that will likely have negative consequences. Ultimately, whether I am talking to kids or adults, we end up agreeing that we prevent the balloon from popping by releasing the air inside—if not all of it, at least some of it. In therapy, sometimes the goal is to prevent the pop by sharing our feelings with the clinician.

Whether you have someone in your life you can talk to or not, therapy could still be a valuable tool to gain new insight and perspective. It may also help you heal from previous emotional hurts, grow beyond an unfortunate experience, or do both. A clinician might make observations or share insights that you were not aware of, causing you to experience an aha moment. Hopefully, a person's decision to seek treatment helps them get to a healthier space, emotionally and mentally. When we're in a better, healthier place, those around us will also benefit. The more we heal ourselves, the better our relationships will be, the better able we are to help others, and the greater the amount of peace and joy we'll likely experience.

WHAT IS THERAPY?

Mental health therapy could be described as a time when a licensed clinician or counselor attempts to assess and treat those struggling with mental, emotional, environmental, or relational challenges. Hopefully, meaningful and positive changes will occur as new strategies and interventions are developed. Anyone, if they so desire, can benefit from having somewhere they can go to help process their personal challenges. Being in a therapy session is a great place to express your deepest thoughts and personal experiences without feeling like someone is judging you or about to condemn and criticize you.

Let me also take a moment to say what therapy *is not*. Therapy is not a magic pill. You don't have a few sessions and then get handed a guarantee you've obtained the results you desired. A large part of effective therapy is the effort that each client is willing to put into treatment.

The progress that a person makes in therapy can be greatly

influenced by what they do in between sessions. Are they attempting to use what they're learning in treatment? Are they changing their thoughts or behaviors in ways that show progress? Are they going in a positive direction that will hopefully lead to a long-lasting change? For example, if I want to get in great shape, I may decide to hire a personal trainer. However, let's say I can only afford to work with them once a week. This could be very beneficial for me. But if I truly want outstanding results, I should probably take the information they're giving me and find ways to work out on my own in between our sessions. Using the personal trainer *and* finding ways to work out on my own increases the likelihood that I'll get the results I'm striving for, perhaps even sooner than I'd planned.

I believe that whether it's individual, couples, or family therapy, the efforts and actions taking place outside of the therapist's office can often play just as big a role as what happens during the session.

DIFFERENT TYPES OF THERAPY

Unbeknownst to most people, there are actually quite a few types of therapy—sometimes referred to as *theoretical orientations*—a clinician may use when working with clients. The theoretical orientation is the particular therapeutic framework, perspective, or concept a mental health professional has been trained in to help, better understand, treat, or provide interventions for the client. It's also very common that a clinician or therapist will use more than one orientation, therefore adopting what's called an *eclectic approach* (drawing from a variety of therapeutic approaches in order to discover which treatment may work best for a specific individual).

Determining the treatment strategy to use comes down to several factors, including what the clinician has experience with or has been trained in, and what they believe may be most beneficial for the client or the client's diagnosis. Some of the more common approaches include psychodynamic therapy, humanistic therapy, and cognitive behavioral therapy. Below I've listed additional options you may have heard of before, or never knew existed:

- Mindfulness-based therapy
- Eye movement desensitization and reprocessing (EMDR)
- Marriage and family therapy
- Group therapy
- Reality therapy
- Animal-assisted therapy
- Exposure therapy
- Expressive arts therapy (including dance movement therapy, art therapy, music therapy, and play therapy)

There are many more than these listed, and typically a therapist will state on their website or in their brochure what theoretical orientation (or orientations) they use. You can also ask what specific techniques they practice or have experience with, in addition to researching them for yourself.

If you or someone you know is seriously thinking about going to therapy, there are some factors you should consider when looking for a clinician. What are the issues or challenges you want to address? Do you need to see someone who specializes in a specific area? Do you prefer a male or female therapist, or someone older or younger? Some minorities seek a therapist of the same race because they feel they will be better understood. This isn't necessarily true, but clients have that right and should be comfortable with the person providing therapy. A person seeking treatment should also consider what they can afford, if they do or do not have insurance, or if the insurance will cover enough of the fee. Of course, paying out of pocket is always an option, if one has the money. Other factors include the days and times that you are available and can commit to attending sessions on a regular basis.

Deciding to go to therapy can be challenging for anyone. It requires the vulnerability, honesty, and even strength to say, "I need help, and I'm willing to take steps to make it happen." We all have challenges or challenging periods, but it can be extremely beneficial if we are able to acknowledge the times when we need outside support.

A therapy session should feel nonthreatening. There should be a certain ease and comfort level present throughout the environment and session. The client should feel that the office or therapeutic setting is a safe space—safe to be open, safe to be vulnerable, safe to disclose, and safe from being judged. Confidentiality, as well as its limitations, should be clearly communicated too. Much of the responsibility for creating this supportive and nurturing environment falls on the clinician. In addition to creating a safe space for my clients, I make every effort to truly understand what my clients are going through and how I may be of service to them.

As the therapist, it's extremely important for me to try to ask the right questions, especially during the initial session. These questions not only allow me to gain valuable information about the client's situation and their past but may also provide them with an opportunity to look inside themselves as they respond. Oftentimes, I feel like a private investigator interviewing a witness while trying to solve a crime. I'm looking for pieces to a puzzle that will assist me in creating as clear an image as possible. The more pieces I have, the better I can understand their situation. Based on their responses, I can then create a picture that allows both of us to understand not only what the true issues are but how to work collaboratively on creating a path toward resolving them and healing.

Please know that no one therapist is perfect for everyone (as I pointed out with my own story). Hearing about a clinician who has done some amazing things does not mean you will have the same outcome. Therefore, be willing to seek out a therapist who is a good fit for you and/or your loved ones.

BARRIERS TO SEEKING TREATMENT

Doubt and fear are the great enemies of knowledge.

—James Allen

For some, deciding to go to therapy might be difficult for reasons other than money, insurance complications, or accessibility. Even with many struggling with depression, anxiety, and stress, and so much uncertainty in our world, there are still plenty of people who are reluctant to consider treatment. There are a variety of reasons an individual, a family, or a couple refuses to give therapy a try. There are those who feel like their situation isn't really a "big deal." Others try to convince themselves that they can handle their issues by saying, "I got this," which may or may not be true. Perhaps an individual can successfully navigate whatever personal challenges they are experiencing. But on the other hand, this may just be wishful thinking.

Sometimes people minimize or flat-out deny that their situation is a problem. Our egos might tell us we don't need anyone's help. Hip-hop recording artist, producer, and entrepreneur Jay-Z has been known to say, "You can't heal what you won't reveal." There's a lot of truth in these words. There is also the old saying "Time heals all wounds." Now I do agree that time can help the healing process. However, saying "all wounds" might be a bit of an overstatement. Often, to heal our broken places—our emotional or mental pain—we must first be willing to admit that they exist. In other words, you can't fix what you don't acknowledge is in need of repair.

Then there are those with strong religious beliefs who are reluctant, or even completely against, meeting with a licensed mental health professional. They may believe that whatever it is they're going through is "God's will" or "in God's hands." Some of their beliefs may lead them to feel that the best way to deal with a difficult issue is to pray and trust that "God will fix it." Perhaps, if one's faith is strong enough, "God" will indeed "fix it." I have no issue with those who have a certain faith or who believe in a supreme being. I find it can often be very healthy to believe in something much greater or larger than ourselves, especially if it promotes healing, gives us a greater sense of peace, and helps us overcome a difficult situation.

However, I also believe we all have gifts, and for some, these gifts may include helping others with their challenges by using their ability to empathize, listen, understand, and guide. These gifts, many believe, are given to people by God (or the universe, or whatever supreme being one believes in) in order for them to serve others; these people include clinicians, teachers, coaches, ministers, and neighbors. Positive messages, helpful messengers, and opportunities that promote healing and growth can come from a variety of people and resources.

I've had some clients admit to being scared to go to therapy because of the pain that may be brought up during a session. They were fearful that talking about past experiences may result in reliving some past trauma and possibly cause some sort of emotional meltdown, leaving them in a worse state than when they arrived. It was during these times that I focused on calming my clients' fears and assisting them with gaining a better understanding of how treatment works and what the goals of therapy are, while hopefully convincing them that they are in an environment where their feelings and emotional well-being are major priorities.

One final reason why people may be reluctant to seek treatment is the continued stigma around mental health. Here we are, in the twenty-first century, and many people still believe that going to therapy means there is something wrong with them. These individuals may make statements such as "I don't need to go see a therapist, because I'm not crazy."

In recent years, thanks to news segments, podcasts, movies, and television, as well as actors, athletes, and politicians (and possibly including people we may know personally) sharing their decisions to get help, much of the stigma around mental health treatment appears to be significantly decreasing. There was a time when most would not dare to admit that they see a therapist; however, I've seen multiple instances where people practically brag or boast that they see their clinician on a regular basis. Unfortunately, this tendency is more likely seen with White people than with minorities, and more commonly seen with women than men—a topic I will dive into later in this book.

WHY PEOPLE GO TO THERAPY

Obviously, there are many reasons why a person might decide to go to therapy. Typically, it means that they are struggling with effectively managing their current situation, their thoughts about a situation, or the emotions that arise as a result. Sometimes a person can feel overwhelmed and unable to determine what to do about their circumstances. Some start therapy because of the suggestion, recommendation, or urging of a doctor, teacher, friend, or family member. I've had clients tell me they wanted a therapist because they didn't feel there was anyone in their life they could turn to without fearing judgment or criticism. I have also worked with those who were mandated by the courts to attend therapy (which includes individual or family treatment). This could be due to significant family disputes, anger issues, abuse, and concerns about custody or visitation between two separated or divorced parents. Then there are those who seek treatment because they are either desperate to make significant and positive changes in their life, or those who simply don't know what else to do.

Once a client has begun working with a licensed mental health professional, more detailed and specific reasons usually emerge as to what needs to be addressed. Some of the more common motives, challenges, and diagnoses that I've noticed include one of or a combination of the following: depression; anxiety; posttraumatic stress disorder; attention deficit hyperactivity disorder; difficulties managing moods/emotions; thoughts of or attempts at suicide; self-injurious behavior such as cutting; grief and loss issues; addiction; relationship conflicts; trauma; feeling stuck; feeling damaged or broken; significant life changes; sexual identity concerns; problems adjusting; being a victim of abuse; a desire for healing, new personal insights, healthier connections with others, or inner peace; feelings of uncertainty; struggles with various fears (real or imagined); family-of-origin issues; intimacy/sexual problems; and low self-esteem. Despite the many items mentioned above, this list in no way covers every diagnosis, situation, or condition leading a person to sit down with a therapist.

Whatever challenges you, a client, a friend, or a family member may be experiencing, please know that sometimes things take time to change. This means you may need to be patient with the process and, more importantly, with yourself. It is also beneficial to be consistent and maintain a sustained effort. But no matter how difficult or how long it may take, I firmly believe change is always possible. When a bone in our body is broken, if it's set correctly, it will grow back even stronger than it was before. I think this can also be true for us emotionally and mentally.

Whether we choose to see a mental health professional or not, there will always be times in our lives when we feel the need to do what we can in order to experience more happiness and a greater overall sense of well-being.

OUR WORST ENEMIES: OUR THOUGHTS, ACTIONS, AND BEHAVIORS

When a client comes to my office, I must first conduct what's called an assessment. This is a time in which I learn what is bringing them in to see me and ask, "How may I serve you?" My goal is to gain an understanding of their situation as they share their story (or the story they have been telling themselves) and their struggle. I also discover who they are, what they think of themselves, how they see their situation, and what interventions they have previously attempted to address the issue. How we view our dilemmas can become very consuming when we repeatedly think, overthink, obsess, and worry about so many things, especially those things we feel we have limited or no control over.

Through my observations, I've learned that how we perceive our circumstances tends to significantly impact our thoughts and emotions. Many times, our perceptions are based on unmet expectations. This typically occurs when something we desire doesn't turn out the way we wanted it to. Examples could include not getting the job we wanted, or getting a job that turns out to be a terrible fit for us. As a matter of fact, I've had clients whose work environments were so toxic that it was creating not only emotional stress but also physical stress. Many of us have also found ourselves in a relationship that does not match the picture we had in our head of how it was supposed to look. We can become consumed with thoughts of disappointment that our lives are not the way we envisioned, which leads us to experience anxiety or depression as well as a variety of other emotions such as panic, frustration, and anger—feelings we try to avoid. We start comparing ourselves to others (and social media makes this all too easy). Some begin to feel that life is not fair. Once consumed with these thoughts, we continue to focus on these unmet expectations over and over. I encourage my clients and friends to keep in mind that what you feed your mind—what you focus on—tends to grow. So be aware and be careful. What you focus on expands.

Many clients who come to see me are overwhelmed about an aspect of their life. This is demonstrated when an individual cannot seem to relinquish toxic thoughts that get replayed in their minds. If we remain in certain negative emotional states for extended periods of time, we risk being overtaken by their adverse effects. Hanging on to a state of mind that produces anger, jealousy, fear, anxiety, grief, or sadness for too long can produce harmful effects not only on ourselves but on those around us. This can lead to some of the diagnoses mentioned earlier, such as anxiety disorder, various forms of depression, and panic attacks, or they can cause us to consider hurting ourselves (emotionally or physically) and possibly others.

We all have stories that we tell ourselves about our lives and who we are. There are those of us who have been victimized, accused, or treated unfairly. Sometimes we're facing situations where we feel like there's no way out or we will never be able to overcome past experiences. Due to our own limited thinking, we may find ourselves unable to become the individuals we want to be and therefore struggle to have the lives we desire.

What are the stories you've been telling yourself about you and your life? Is your life really hopeless, or will you ultimately be triumphant? If you are a therapist or provide some other type of emotional support for others, what is the narrative you're hearing from your clients? What are the stories your friends or family members have been telling themselves repeatedly? Whether you are aware of this or not, our brain and our ego always want us to be *right*. Our brain and our ego will search high and low for the evidence to support whatever beliefs we currently have. If you believe you're unattractive and unworthy of love, guess what? Your brain and ego will come up with reasons why this is true. If you believe you will never get a high-paying job you enjoy, then the reasons why it's not possible will pop into your head. I've learned that once people believe a thing to be true, it will be demonstrated by their actions and behaviors—whether those actions are positive, negative, or somewhere in between. Our behaviors often follow or demonstrate our beliefs.

We often believe that we're trapped in our situations, when in reality, we're often prisoners of our own limiting thoughts. Because of our conditioning, ignorance, and insecurities, there are times when these beliefs cause us to miss out on the possible solutions and even blessings that are actually present.

READY TO WORK?

When a person is struggling with mental health issues but truly wants things to get better, they have to be ready to work and sincerely be willing to make the effort for their life to be improved. This is not always easy, and even deciding to go to therapy can be difficult. But if an individual is able to realize it's worth it to at least try therapy *and* muster the courage to make an appointment, there are *three primary steps* that will likely pave the way to a greater chance of success while achieving the identified therapeutic goals.

1. *Being aware of or admitting that there is an issue that needs to be addressed.*

Many times in individual, couples, and family therapy, someone in the room does not believe that there is a problem or that something needs to be changed or addressed. I've had couples sitting directly in front of me, and someone will say that whatever perceived issues their partner has identified as a problem, they don't view it as such. Some have even suggested that their significant other is the problem, or the only one experiencing an issue. They think it's the other person who needs to change. I've had clients demonstrate or disclose addictions, whether it's marijuana, pornography, or even shopping; however, they believe it's not a problem because they are in complete control of every aspect of their lives. If a person isn't willing to acknowledge their areas of weakness, areas where growth is needed, or how they are negatively impacting their life and their relationships, change is not likely to happen. In Alcoholics Anonymous, the first of the twelve steps is acknowledging or admitting you have a problem you are struggling to manage. However, once we take ownership and are truly willing to look deeply at what needs to be done, we are on our way to making change.

2. *Truly wanting to change.*

When a person has decided they can no longer deal with a situation or something about themselves, the odds of them doing something different increase. Mind you, these are typically clients who are tired of feeling overwhelmed or tired of feeling the heavy weight of whatever it is they've been carrying. These individuals may feel like they can't go any lower or are basically fed up with the way things have been. At this point, they have likely gained both the strength and the motivation that, up until now, were absent. Hopefully, they believe they are now able to produce enough leverage to make positive changes.

I've shared with clients and friends that people typically change for one of several reasons. First, they truly can't take the misery anymore. They are ready for their lives to be different, if not better. Perhaps they've had an aha moment. In this case, they may have been exposed to or learned something they were previously unaware of and are now ready to use this information to alter their life for the better.

Another reason an individual may want to bring change into their life is they feel a strong need to change for someone else. There are many people who, because of their love or desire to please a loving partner, family member, or friend, will make change happen. Some of us won't do for ourselves what we are willing to do for our loved ones. For them, we will make whatever personal sacrifices are necessary.

Finally, I've seen people who are ready for change when they've experienced a powerful moment that can't be ignored, where it feels like life has come along and simply punched them in the face—hard! I'm talking about life circumstances that shake them to their core and cause them to reevaluate everything they've been doing up until this point. Perhaps they're in the middle of a crisis, such as being on the verge of losing a wonderful relationship. Maybe their health condition has taken a turn for the worse and they are now forced to heed their doctor's advice. Maybe they have lost something they simply can't get back, like a loved one who has passed, a once-in-a-lifetime job, or a life-changing opportunity. Maybe a lack of motivation or self-discipline has resulted in significant financial difficulties. Or maybe some form of addiction (drugs, alcohol, sex, gambling, shopping, etc.) has caused irreparable damage.

Regardless of why a client or individual wants things to be different, change is often not only inevitable but also necessary for personal healing and growth.

3. *Being willing to work.*

The third and final step that can go a long way toward therapy being successful is the client's understanding that they will be required to put forth the necessary effort to obtain the results they desire. They must be willing to do some things that perhaps they didn't do or didn't consider doing before in order to produce change.

Sometimes people come into my office expressing that they want something better for themselves, their relationships, or their lives. That sounds great. We should all want to find ways to create the best life possible for ourselves. It's important to continue striving to evolve and grow in various areas of our lives. The question I then have to ask is "Are you truly ready to put in the work?" By *work*, I mean doing things differently than they've done before. Are they ready to think differently, consider other perspectives, make other choices, take different actions, or completely add or eliminate a behavior (if realistically possible)? Part of the work may include reading books (that may help with reaching goals), considering the perspective of others, practicing patience, practicing forgiveness, showing self-restraint, being more open-minded, being respectful of others, demonstrating grace, using self-care interventions, or simply doing things they previously didn't want to do, thought they didn't need to do, or believed would be too difficult.

It's usually much easier to say what you want than to

actually create what you want. Anyone can say they want to look great, start a business, write a book, quit smoking, purchase a home, or get a college degree, but to obtain those goals a person must be willing to take action or take risks even if it means being in uncomfortable situations. Making a positive shift in our lives can be challenging, but I don't recall anyone ever saying doing what's right, good, and beneficial is supposed to be easy.

BARRIERS TO INNER PEACE

Many of us (in therapy or not) truly seek a happy life, which usually includes the desire for inner peace. I describe inner peace as a feeling of contentment and appreciation for one's life and what they have. For me, inner peace also comes with a sense of calmness, fulfillment, joy, and acceptance of the aspects of life that we cannot change. I'm sure you may have your own definition of inner peace, but that's typically what I strive for.

Having inner peace is definitely a worthy goal, and therapy can be a part of achieving it. However, there are so many things that can prevent one from experiencing the peace we so often crave. Barriers that hinder us from having more overall peace and happiness in life may be the result of being overwhelmed and weighed down by any of the following: excessive worry, blaming others, feeling overwhelmed by tasks, frequent arguing, lack of certainty or security, being overly focused on achievement, displaying excessive anger or being unable to control one's anger, not feeling valued, holding on to resentment, judging others harshly or unnecessarily, lust, feeling separated from others, always rushing or in a hurry, bitterness, unresolved trauma, lack of self-discipline, guilt, frequently feeling under pressure, being unappreciative, feeling fatigued, feeling burned out, obsession or being obsessed, engaging in fighting/violence, desiring what belongs to another/coveting, insecurities, being reluctant or refusing to care for others, difficulty with surrendering or letting things go (situations, expectations, or people), having to be right, greed, pain (physical, mental, emotional, or spiritual), ignorance, loneliness, and living in a constant state of fear.

This, of course, is not an exhaustive list but simply the barriers I most often see in my office and in our world. If a person truly wants peace, they must be willing to let go of the obstacles described, change their mindset, and then change their behaviors. At the very least, they must find and use healthier ways to address these challenges.

CHAPTER 2

Lessons Learned About Anxiety and Depression

The primary cause of unhappiness is never the situation but your thoughts about it. Be aware of the thoughts you are thinking.

—Eckhart Tolle

Years ago, I was working as a therapist at a residential facility for children and adolescents with significant psychiatric, behavioral, or neurological issues. It was a hospital setting, and often the kids would not only go to school there but remain anywhere from one month to well over a year. I had just returned to work in December after having a hernia operation and was experiencing one of the worst bouts of depression in my entire life.

Allow me to give you some background on my situation at the time. I'd been living in Atlanta at that point for about three years and had not yet formed any kind of social network. With no close friends and no romantic relationship, I spent most of my weekends either hanging out at Barnes & Noble or watching television. I did have a couple of coworkers who I hung out with from time to time outside of my job, but that was a rarity. More often than not, I found myself alone. Now don't get me wrong; there is nothing wrong with being alone. But I was struggling with loneliness. I was also struggling with crushing burnout. Working at this facility with so many kids displaying so many challenging issues (from emotional instability to physical aggression) had me questioning how much longer I could endure this. I had only been there a year and a half, but realistically, it was probably six months too long. As a result, I often found myself becoming emotional, stressed, and tearful as I sat in my apartment alone. To top it off, I had been off work for a week recovering from my surgery and had to go through the ordeal by myself. Grocery shopping, preparing meals, and dealing with the pain while my body was trying to recover from the procedure were very difficult and depressing to do alone.

The first day back at work was brutal. It took me until the middle of the day to muster up the energy to see even one child in a therapy session. I eventually did, but it wasn't easy. At some point during the early evening hours, I simply couldn't take it anymore and left an hour earlier than normal.

When I look back on that time, what's interesting is the fact that it never occurred to me to seek out a therapist of my own to address what I was dealing with. To be honest, I'm not really sure why I didn't. Perhaps I had some sort of macho mentality where I thought I could handle whatever I was dealing with on my own. Maybe, since I spent so much time with young people who needed therapy, I, as an adult, thought I should be able to navigate my way out of whatever mental state I was in. If I could do it all over again, I believe I would've made an effort to find a therapist of my own and work through whatever it was I was dealing with at the time.

I will say there was a happy ending to this emotional and challenging day. You see, while driving home from work that evening, I decided to stop at Whole Foods, and without going into too much detail, I met a woman (in the produce aisle!) who would ultimately become my best friend and wife. That's quite a story in itself, but I'll have to save that for another time. (It does go to show you that when you're struggling, an amazing breakthrough could be right around the corner, literally.)

My situation illustrates that anxiety or, in my case, depression can happen to anybody at any time, and often does. In my experience as a marriage and family therapist, the conditions commonly referred to as *depression* and *anxiety* have been the primary reasons why adults in particular have come to me seeking therapy. Most of us at some point experience some degree of one or both. Even though depression and anxiety are normal human struggles, the big concern is remaining in either of these states too long. If we do, it's possible to become so overwhelmed with sadness that it grows and becomes some form of diagnosable depression—or we worry for so long and intensely that the anxiety feels like it's simply too difficult to manage or let go of. When either of these emotional states impede our ability to function and negatively affect our everyday lives and our interactions with others, then it's time to consider getting some help.

In this chapter we will be focusing on these two potentially harmful diagnoses, in addition to trying to better understand and treat them.

WHAT IS ANXIETY?

There are plenty of sources out there that provide thorough definitions for anxiety. But to keep things simple, I will describe anxiety as intense and consistent worrying about situations and what's going on in one's life.

When we experience anxiety, we tend to be stressed. In my therapy sessions, I've heard clients express challenging thoughts and feelings that make them believe their lives are completely out of their control. Like many of us, they often place a significant amount of emphasis on their expectations, hopes, or desired outcomes. When important things are not going the way we would like them to, we can easily find ourselves stressed and swimming in feelings of anxiousness.

MANAGING ANXIETY, INCLUDING MY OWN

There was a period in my life when I used to spend a significant amount of time worrying about my future. It was very common for me to say things like "What if I don't achieve this goal?" "What if I don't have enough money?" "What if they don't hire me?" "What if this physical ailment is something really serious?" or "What if I'm destined to be alone for the rest of my life?" I can't tell you how many times questions like these replayed in my head over and over again. Fortunately, I was able to learn the value of being in the present moment and faithfully trusting that things will ultimately be okay. Now please don't think that I've mastered the art of a worry-free life. I assure you that this is definitely not the case. I frequently have internal conversations with myself, speak words of faith and encouragement to myself, talk things through with my wife, and pray when I feel overly concerned about something. However, I truly believe I have made significant progress when it comes to preventing worry from taking over my thoughts.

There were many tools I used to help me from drowning in excessive worry. I read a variety of self-improvement and spiritual growth books (and still do). I listened to advice from those sharing their opinions in workshops, audiobooks, and podcasts. Over the years I've watched quite a few motivational and inspirational videos on YouTube and attended seminars and trainings focusing on being or becoming a better version of myself, including being someone who deals with difficult situations better.

About seven years ago, I began practicing meditation and yoga on a daily basis. I noticed how often various challenges in my life ultimately were resolved, often resulting in an even better outcome than I could have imagined. As much as I possibly could, I also tried to read, say, and remind myself of "The Serenity Prayer": *God grant me the serenity to accept the things I cannot change, the courage to change the things that I can, and the wisdom to know the difference.*[1]

I demonstrated acceptance by acknowledging the things in life that I have no control over (both in the past and present), and I've tried to focus on the parts of a given situation that I could change. Using these interventions helped me not only manage my own anxiety and stress but also better serve my clients. On many occasions, I would find myself sharing with clients what has worked for me and exploring whether these things would benefit them as well.

I realize that minimizing or eliminating anxiety is much easier said than done. How many times have we heard someone say, "Just have faith," "Everything will be okay," or "There's nothing to worry about. It'll all work out in the end"? However, despite how challenging it may be, we all have a choice. As a matter of fact, every day we make decisions when it comes to anxiety and stress. We get to decide whether or not we will try our best to effectively manage whatever is stressing us out. We get to decide if we are going to embrace hope and faith, or if we are going to do nothing but worry, doubt, and live in fear. It's usually an either-or decision. We can choose to live in faith or fear, but it's difficult to live in both at the same time.

When we're excessively worrying, we're likely feeding our fears and allowing them to gain more strength and control over us and the situation. I've learned through my experiences, as well as those of my clients, that sometimes the fear is that we may end up feeling ashamed or embarrassed. We fear we may fail. We fear what others will think. We fear not having control. Or we simply have a fear of the unknown.

I believe the reason fear is so prevalent in our world, in our society, and within each of us is that we long for security and certainty. And yet there are some benefits to learning to embrace the unknown. Accepting that there are always various outcomes can actually be exciting. I know movies do not depict real life; however, we tend to enjoy them more when we don't know what's about to happen next. We are then able to share in the experiences of the characters on the screen. Maybe it's not such a bad idea to think of our lives as an adventure to be experienced and enjoyed even if we're not 100 percent sure of the outcome.

Finally, let's not underestimate the role that faith can have in managing anxiety. For clarity's sake, when I say faith, I'm not necessarily referring to religion (but it definitely can be). I'm referring to a belief that things can and will get better. Faith is often about having a belief in something that currently might not be known or visible. Faith is continuing to have hope. Faith is also believing in something greater than yourself and trusting that things will work out.

THE BOXES WE CARRY

There is a metaphor I often use with clients, friends, and students as it relates to managing stress and anxiety. (I'll be sharing a very similar metaphor in the self-care chapter.) It's very difficult for many of us to get through our lives without experiencing stress. It might be helpful to think of a stressful situation as being represented by a box. Now think about us having multiple boxes, each a different size and weight. We are all trying to move forward through life while carrying these boxes. Some of us have more boxes, and some of us have fewer boxes. Overall, we are simply trying to manage our load. Continuing with this metaphor, I've seen clients struggle while carrying only one or two small boxes that to some would be a breeze to handle. But I understand that we're not all built the same; we all don't have the same strength or stamina. But we *do* all have to know how much of a load, or how many boxes, we can carry before we become overwhelmed, stressed, or anxious. Sometimes this means deciding which boxes we need to put down, at least for now, allowing us the opportunity to rest and gain renewed strength. Then, when we're ready, we can pick the boxes up again and continue navigating down the road that is our life. There may even be a box or two that we need to put down and never pick up again.

Despite how challenging it can be to deal with stress, some stress is often necessary for personal growth (as long as the stress does not become overwhelming and debilitating). Most people who've accomplished significant goals have struggled. Along their journey they had to push themselves through whatever challenges that were standing before them. As a result, they became stronger and more skilled. The obstacles are what caused growth to happen, enabling them to achieve their goal. People don't typically go to the gym with a desire to get strong by lifting extremely light weights. Becoming stronger often involves lifting enough weight to be a challenge, where the repeated resistance pushes and strains the muscles, causing them to grow and get stronger.

We even see how the struggle is necessary in nature, whether it's a caterpillar developing its wings by pushing on the inside of a cocoon, or a baby chick building up its muscles by pecking at the inside of its shell. These are necessary struggles that prepare these creatures for their future.

One additional thing to consider: when it comes to anxiety, no matter how much we worry about something, worrying alone will not change a thing. The outcome of most situations will likely only change because of the actions we decide to take and the thoughts we decide to have (or let go of).

WHAT IS DEPRESSION?

While living in Burbank, California, I remember going through a very challenging period in my life. So many evenings I found myself sitting in my small studio apartment completely alone and wishing I had someone to talk to or go somewhere with. I often spent many weekends overcoming my boredom by trying to find something to do besides sitting on my couch looking at the TV or reading a book. Not that I mind doing those things. Quite the contrary! I do enjoy those activities, but the real issue was that I was extremely lonely *and* felt alone. I had yet to form any significant friendships or close relationships. I would try to call my friends back home in Chicago or a few I had in other cities, but more often than not, they were not available, so I found myself leaving messages and hoping for a returned call. I tried not to reach out too often because I didn't want to be annoying, but there were a lot of weekends where I did not speak to a single person from Friday night until Monday morning (when I returned to work). I really struggled with the feeling of being separated, alone, and lonely. I know now, looking back, that not feeling connected to others was making me feel depressed. It was quite painful, and I'm sure I'm not the only one who has experienced this situation, feeling overwhelmed with waves of sadness. It was during this time (and others as well) that I personally learned what some degree of depression can feel like and the challenges it presents when trying to manage the feeling.

I've had many clients struggle with anxiety; however, I've encountered significantly more who are dealing with one of the various levels of depression. Depression, likely more common and undiagnosed than we may realize, is a serious condition that impairs one's ability to function, in addition to impacting how a person feels and views their life, their situation, or themselves. Symptoms can include feeling sad, hopeless, and pessimistic. A person dealing with depression may lack motivation, have low energy, or struggle significantly to do tasks that are common or necessary for daily living. Additional symptoms may be a change of appetite (not being hungry or eating significantly more than usual), difficulty falling asleep, sleeping too much, feelings of low self-worth, or questioning whether they want to continue living or not.

As I stated previously, whenever an individual is seriously considering suicide or attempting it, they should get help immediately. Going to the nearest hospital, calling 911, or calling the Suicide and Crisis Lifeline at 988 are actions that may save a person's life.

The Depression Spectrum

I view depression and various other diagnoses as if they are on a spectrum. A person could be on the far left, where their depression hovers around being a more manageable type of sadness that most of us experience at some point in our lives. Then there is the far right of the spectrum, where depression is debilitating or paralyzing, possibly even producing thoughts of suicide or suicide attempts. Individuals on this end of the spectrum are often struggling with deeply rooted issues, such as severe trauma, being totally overwhelmed by one's situation, a family history of depression, and ongoing chronic illness, just to name a few.

There are, of course, other triggers that may cause a person to feel depressed. In my personal and professional life, I've witnessed how individuals who feel separated or disconnected from others have significant amounts of emotional pain. This was a big part of what I was experiencing while living in LA. Now let's look at other possible causes and contributing factors that can lead to depression.

Social Media, Society-Based Success,
and Our Craving for Stuff

Unfortunately, today's modern technology (in this case social media) has provided yet another doorway to depression. Former President Theodore Roosevelt said, "Comparison is the thief of joy."[2] There is definitely some truth in this statement when I think about the many clients I've had, of various ages, who spend a significant amount of time comparing themselves to others they see on social media. They look at what some people claim to have accomplished and compare that to what they have or haven't done. Some look at romantic relationships on social media and envy what they see because they don't have someone to call their own. Social media also makes it easy to compare one's appearance to that of others online. This may lead them to question their own looks, to be jealous of others, to criticize themselves for what they see as flaws or imperfections, and to feel inadequate.

But it's not just those we see on social media who can cause us to question ourselves and our self-worth. There are other people in society and in our everyday lives who contribute (knowingly or unknowingly) to making us feel like we don't measure up or are not successful until a certain goal has been met. Those who may be adding pressure or stress to our lives could include our parents, people we believe are our friends, partners or significant others, coworkers, and the media (television, films, magazines, advertisements). For better or worse, we often find ourselves seeking validation from others. This should come from within—meaning, we should really be striving to find the good and positive that exist inside each of us and allow that to shape how we view ourselves.

The constant bombardment of images on television, social media, and magazines also reminds us of all the things we don't have but, according to corporations and big businesses, we need. We are made to feel we must have the latest, trendiest, most expensive item in order to impress people and feel good about ourselves.

The pressure to have, to succeed, or to measure up to the expectations of others has significantly contributed to the high levels of depression in both my adolescent and adult clients. When materialistic desires aren't being met, many people become stressed and depressed because they have in their minds a picture of what they believe success looks like (and anything less than that is failure). I wish that people's definition of success could be broader and incorporate other things, like having people we love in our lives, good health, a sense of gratitude, serving others in a positive way, developing a legacy of love and compassion, and simply being happy. There's nothing inherently wrong with having big goals and dreams or pursuing the finer things in life. However, if trying to obtain "stuff" or trying to meet someone else's definition of success jeopardizes a person's emotional, mental, physical, or spiritual health, it's probably not worth it.

PRODUCING CHANGE

Both professionally and personally, I have seen times when symptoms associated with depression, anxiety, or other mental health disorders have been reduced, managed, or even eliminated. How is this done? Well, as you can imagine, there is no clear, undefeated way of curing these conditions. Typically, different interventions work for different people. What may work for one person may not do anything for the next.

If we truly want to change, grow, and heal, it's extremely beneficial to be open-minded. One must not only be open and willing to consider the many tools or interventions that may help, but also be aware that change takes time and always requires effort. Whether it's a client or you who is struggling with anxiety or depression, if you want positive and meaningful change, you will have to start by taking action. This means being willing to do *something* differently in order to get different and, hopefully, positive results.

Regardless of whether it's depression or anxiety, there are several areas I typically like to explore with my clients. I prefer to spend time learning about and helping them with two things: first, their awareness of the thoughts or beliefs they have about themselves, their life, and their situation (including the words they speak and the beliefs they've attached to them), and second, their willingness to take action. During this time, I am also looking at their barriers and triggers that may be interfering with making the necessary changes or taking much-needed action.

Now let's spend a little time breaking down each of these areas and the role they may play when it comes to treating anxiety and depression.

OUR THOUGHTS AND BELIEFS

Disturbances come from within, from our own perceptions.

—Marcus Aurelius

In many ways, we are all like gardeners for our thoughts. As gardeners, we play a significant role in determining what we plant in our yard, what is put into the soil, and how much care, time, and attention we intend to give the plants. Like gardeners, we need to be aware of what we've planted or allowed someone else to plant in our minds. It is up to us to tend this garden on a regular basis in order to produce positive results— our harvest. We must also weed out the stuff we don't want— the things that are making it difficult for our garden to thrive. It's up to us to make sure that what we're trying to grow is getting enough water and the right amount of sunlight, while also addressing things that could cause problems, such as weeds, animals, and insects. If we don't address these things, they will likely have negative consequences that we will then be forced to deal with later.

If we fail to manage our thoughts and our beliefs about ourselves, we provide an opportunity for toxic or negative beliefs to rule. It's extremely important to be aware of the harmful, negative stories we repeatedly tell ourselves about our lives and who we are. It also becomes increasingly likely that these types of thoughts will negatively affect others, especially those we love and influence the most. At the very least, these thoughts will hinder us from experiencing inner peace and a greater sense of happiness.

So how does one begin nurturing and taking care of their thoughts, or mental garden? For starters, if we truly want change to occur, we must first be open and honest with ourselves and what our issues, patterns, or tendencies are. In other words, we must start with awareness. Many people are reluctant to take an honest look within and acknowledge their fears, their pain, their past, their brokenness, their trauma, and what parts of their lives need to change. If a client is unwilling to do that, then as a therapist it becomes very difficult to reach the desired outcomes or achieve significant results.

Hopefully, clients are coming to therapy because they are ready to face their issues head-on. Many people go through their daily lives oblivious to the fact that they have any issues at all, while others prefer to ignore or deny them. These people typically do not seek help let alone a mental health professional. If someone points a concern out to them, they might say, "I'm fine. I'm good. I got this. No problems here." Once we can accept that we have a challenge "to grow through," we can then begin focusing and working on ourselves. Or to paraphrase the lyrics of a Michael Jackson song, we should probably start with the person staring back at us in the mirror.

Monitoring our thoughts and beliefs (especially those that can produce anxiety or feelings of depression) is extremely important. It can provide you with the opportunity to pay attention to how you are currently thinking about yourself, how you are seeing others, and how you are perceiving your current situation (or situations). How are you viewing your traumatic or abusive past? Sometimes we feel like we have an insurmountable problem, when in reality we may just need to view it from a different perspective. Perhaps the perceived adversity is creating opportunities for growth, ultimately producing positive outcomes in our lives. Please keep in mind that just because you don't see the light or a way out of your situation doesn't mean one doesn't exist.

If you close your eyes right now and see nothing but darkness, it doesn't mean you aren't surrounded by light. You have some control to decide what to think about, how long you want to focus on a specific thought, and what action you plan to take (if any). Consider asking yourself empowering questions, such as "What can I learn from the situation?" "Can I reframe or see this matter in a different, less threatening way?" "Is it possible that this challenge can help me evolve into a better version of myself?"

We often demonstrate where we are mentally and emotionally by the words we speak. What we say out loud shows our current thoughts and beliefs. I'm sure there are many people who believe that their words simply reflect what they're feeling on the inside at a given moment, and that can definitely be true. However, it can also be true that the words you've been replaying inside your mind *and then speaking out loud* have contributed to your current emotional state. (I'm excluding those who have much deeper psychological challenges.)

There are many who believe, myself included, that words have the power to both create and destroy, to hurt and heal. For those who hold religious beliefs, there are multiple verses in the Bible that make references to the power of the spoken word.

We should therefore be wary of the negative words and statements we say out loud, especially if we do it often or in ways that make us feel defeated, helpless, anxious, or sad. If we frequently use negative or derogatory words and statements to describe ourselves or our situation, we could actually be making ourselves victims and, without knowing it, taking away our power to effectively overcome our issues.

For example, what if I woke up this morning and immediately thought and then verbalized, "I feel like crap! What's the use of even trying"? What if I repeatedly said these things throughout the morning and into the afternoon? I would go through a significant portion of the day (if not the entire day) feeling poorly, unconfident, and low. After all, *crap* is usually a synonym for garbage or waste. But what if I woke up this morning and said, "I feel strong, healthy, and fantastic!"? In this case, I'll likely have a greater chance of going through the day with my head held high, projecting confidence, and probably looking good too. What a stark contrast in statements. One morning I'm using my words to reinforce feeling crappy and useless, while on another day my words are empowering, lifting me up both mentally and emotionally.

When it comes to assisting a client, supporting a friend, or even trying to maintain a healthy mindset, it's extremely important to be aware of what words are placed after the statement "I am." Instead of making comments like "I am unwanted," "I am unattractive," "I am poor," or "I am not going to succeed," a better way to use these two powerful words would be to say, "I am desired by those who are right for me," "I am good looking," "I am wealthy" (perhaps in ways not solely attached with money or materialism), and "I am going to accomplish my goal and achieve something even better."

I am not saying that simply speaking positive statements about yourself or placing positive words after "I am" will guarantee that the changes you seek will miraculously appear overnight and transforms your life. However, there is value in being aware of how the words you say out loud or to yourself may be impacting your mental health or overall mindset.

The bottom line is that words matter. Whether it's the words you're thinking, saying to yourself, saying to others, listening to or hearing, writing down, reading, singing, or seeing on a regular basis. Words matter so much that they can be one of several keys to positive change and growth. If, however, the words are negative and toxic, they'll likely contribute to keeping us stuck in a life filled with disappointment and pain.

TAKING ACTION TO CREATE CHANGE REQUIRES EFFORT

Have you known someone who often talked about how they wanted to be different or how they wanted their life to be different? Perhaps they talked a lot about wanting to lose weight, but when asked, "Are you working out? Have you changed your diet?" they responded, "No, not yet," or "I plan on starting soon." Maybe for years you've heard a friend or family member talk about their plans to quit smoking, but they never took the first step, let alone sought out some of the many options out there to help quit this habit.

There are people who readily admit that they've endured trauma from their past and have significant emotional issues that need to be dealt with—problems that are producing anxiety or depression. But for some reason, they never seem to be able to make that first appointment to see a licensed therapist. They never take the time to do research or read books that may help them deal with their issues. Plain and simple: if we want to change any aspect of our lives, we can't just talk about the issues; we have to start the process and be disciplined enough to "walk the walk." In other words, take action. However, when you finally decide to put in the effort, please realize that the first step is great, but it's usually not enough. Lasting change requires multiple steps that include being *consistent*. Growth toward a goal is rarely obtained without some degree of regular effort. A person must be willing to strive to think the right thoughts, speak the right words, and take the right actions. Do the work that will get the results you are seeking. Positive change doesn't come without putting in the time (no matter how long it may take) and making the effort (no matter how difficult or hard it may be).

Sometimes doing what's in our best interest may mean stepping outside of our comfort zone and taking the necessary risk to achieve our desired outcome. It may be scary, it may be difficult, but it also may be exactly what's needed.

DIFFICULT CHOICES AND LIFESTYLE CHANGES

Addressing depressive symptoms and anxiety often requires people to do some things differently, which may include altering how one lives their life. Some examples of what I mean are going to see a therapist, making changes in one's diet (eating healthily, reducing sugar intake, etc.), increasing exercise/movement (before beginning any exercise routine, please consult with a doctor, especially if you have concerns about or history of physical health issues), getting better sleep, and reducing or eliminating drugs/alcohol.

In the upcoming chapter on self-care, I spend time discussing more specific interventions that can benefit anyone, including those who are struggling with true psychological diagnoses, such as depression or anxiety. I'll make recommendations for things to do as well as what to avoid in order to better equip you to deal with today's challenges. I'll also discuss the importance of nurturing your mind, your body, and your spirit if you are to become more at peace in the best version of yourself.

At this time, however, I'd like to look at three additional areas to consider when depression or anxiety are present. These are the possible benefits of expressing gratitude, focusing on the well-being of others, and taking medication.

One way to improve your emotional state is simply to take time to identify the things in your life that you're grateful for. There have been times during therapy sessions (based on what's being discussed at the moment) when I'll ask the client to pause and share with me the things in their life they are grateful for. It's a good idea for us all to take a moment to remind ourselves that somewhere in the world (possibly even in our own neighborhoods or families), there is someone who would rather change places with us than deal with what they're going through in their own life. Fortunately, the majority of us have far more blessings and good fortune in our lives than perceived issues or challenges.

As part of my daily meditation, I spend time every morning identifying at least two to three things that I'm thankful for. I strongly believe in not taking things for granted. I even have a few of my college students begin the first class of each week by sharing something good they've experienced lately or something that they're thankful for.

Another idea that I've explored with some clients to help reduce symptoms of depression or anxiety is volunteering (if deemed appropriate, a good fit for the individual, and they're open to it). Volunteering provides people with the opportunity to think about someone other than themselves. Volunteering could provide an opportunity for them to take a break from thinking about their current struggles and instead focus on serving someone else. Most clients do see the possible value in volunteering, and I've had a few who actually wanted to do it; however, they typically indicate not having the time. On a few occasions, clients have at least agreed to become more intentional about doing things for a family member or a friend in need.

In my twenties and early thirties, I spent a significant amount of time volunteering with various organizations that included a children's hospital (for terminally ill youth), an animal shelter, and the physical therapy department of a hospital on the North Side of Chicago. Whenever I was at these facilities, my attention was solely focused on doing my job and helping in any way I possibly could. In doing so, whatever I was struggling with was put on the back burner. This was especially true when working at the children's hospital, knowing that some of these kids were dealing with a condition they may not recover from. One truly unfortunate young boy I worked with had been intentionally burned (abused) over 85 to 90 percent of his body. Trust me, when I was with him my concerns of the day paled in comparison.

One final way to treat a variety of mental health issues, including anxiety and depression, is utilizing psychotropic medications. Since I'm not a medical doctor, I strongly recommend that an individual experiencing significant struggles seek out medical care, especially those who are finding it difficult to manage their emotions, thoughts, and actions, or those who feel suicidal or have issues that significantly impact their daily lives in negative and harmful ways. There's a possibility that medication is a legitimate option to consider to help a person who is truly struggling with their diagnosis. Of course, medication should only be administered and monitored by a doctor. This is especially important since all medications are not created equal, can affect different people differently, and could possibly have side effects, creating additional unwanted consequences. A qualified doctor should be able to consider different options for medications, explain how they work, and address any questions the person may have. Once a doctor has identified the correct drug that may benefit the patient, the physician may also strongly encourage them to see, or continue seeing, a therapist as well. Many studies indicate that psychotropic medications along with therapy can be more beneficial than just medication alone.

ACCEPTANCE AND PUSHING THROUGH

Clients have come to me expressing frustration after frustration as they attempt to manage many challenging aspects of their lives. These are often issues that cause people to feel overwhelmed and extremely stressed. Perhaps it's a wife who feels her spouse is trying to control her, a manager who seems hell-bent on making their employees feel useless, an applicant who did not get the job they wanted, or someone who has lost a beloved family member. These are all situations that can be very difficult to manage, but the one thing they have in common is that they make us feel we are not in control of our lives. Feeling we have no control often produces feelings of anxiousness or thoughts leading to depression.

When things happen to us that feel incredibly difficult to deal with, we may need to accept the fact that there are times when all we can do is try—try to move forward and grow through our dilemma. Sometimes working through these challenges means learning to embrace acceptance, or at least trying to. At some point, we are all forced to deal with unfortunate situations. For example, none of us will live forever (at least not in this current physical form), and those whom we love will die as well. Sometimes we may have a goal that we so desperately want, but for whatever reason we are not able to achieve it. Perhaps it will be beneficial for some of us to consider that achieving a goal doesn't have to look exactly the way we imagined. And let's also take the time to appreciate the journey and the opportunities that life presents to us.

Setbacks, disappointments, and coming up short are always a possibility. But it's in our best interest to try to move forward. Clients have told me they were so depressed they couldn't get out of bed. It was during these times I encouraged them to at least figure out what they *could* do, and then go and do that. Maybe it was difficult to get out of bed and go to work. Ask yourself, "Can I go for a walk in the neighborhood?" Can you muster up enough energy to eat something, despite not having an appetite? Can you push yourself to make it to the therapist's office where you may get just what you need for this day, this week, or beyond? The ability to push through is important for personal growth. It's through the struggle that we gain strength.

CHAPTER 3

Lessons Learned About Couples Therapy

As long as we cling to our agendas and our illusions, we do not truly love. Let them be who they are. If they leave, it might be because they were supposed to go.

—Elisabeth Kübler-Ross and David Kessler

In my late twenties, I was in my first truly challenging relationship. At this point, I had been in two previous long-term relationships of about two to three years. In both cases I was involved with wonderful young women whom I cared about. They cared about me, and for the most part, we had some good times. Now, these relationships weren't perfect by any stretch of the imagination, especially considering our ages, our limited life experiences, and our overall emotional intelligence (or lack thereof), but I would still describe them as meaningful and an important part of my past because I believe they helped prepare me to be married. In both instances, the relationships ended when they decided, for different reasons, to break up with me and move on. But even to this day, I am grateful for the time that I had with each. Then came a relationship that was very different and tested me like none I'd had before.

Let me start out by saying that the young lady who presented these relational challenges wasn't a bad person at all. She was actually attractive, sweet, and kind. However, despite her positive traits, I had never been in a relationship where I argued as frequently as I did with her. We didn't argue every day (even though it sometimes felt that way), but it was a few times a week—far more than I had ever experienced with any other girlfriend.

I believe we honestly cared for one another, and we tried to make it work. We'd try to identify what the issues were, as well as apply our own interventions or try to do things differently (as a couple and as individuals). This was the first time I went out and purchased books on relationships (which we often read together) in order to try to address our problems. When I look back, I think a lot of our struggles had to do with the expectations we had for one another as well as the expectations we had for the relationship itself.

Nonetheless, after about eight months, we mutually agreed to break up. I believe at that point we were each tired of the back-and-forth debates and the frustration that often accompanied our conflicts. This was also the first time in my life that the other person wasn't making the decision to end the relationship, leaving me heartbroken.

Although the relationship didn't last long, I don't regret being in it one bit. Our situation challenged me and allowed me to gain a new understanding of what it means to make a relationship work. I also learned that some people are only in our lives for a certain period of time, maybe for a particular reason (perhaps for us to heal or learn a much-needed lesson), as well as the fact that there are people who simply aren't a good fit for us (at least for the long haul). Ultimately, we both went on to find the person whom we would marry and, speaking for myself, to experience a far greater level of compatibility and love.

When doing couples therapy, I'm specifically referring to working with two people who are in an intimate relationship. This may include those who are married, engaged, or dating. I have found that conducting couples therapy sessions can be very interesting, rewarding, and definitely challenging. When you really break it down, partnerships are two people who have come together, who were raised in different households, and who had vastly different life experiences and parents with their own beliefs and expectations they imposed on their children. Those in the relationship could be from different cultures and may have different religious perspectives, thus having their own individual values, morals, and principles. Each has likely developed their own definition of what it means to be in a satisfying relationship. If you really think about it, it's amazing people get together—let alone stay together—at all. Helping couples achieve the goals that brought them to therapy will typically require all three of us to put in some work and be as open-minded as possible if the relationship is going to be made better.

WHY DO COUPLES GO TO THERAPY?

Of course, there are a variety of reasons why a couple may have found themselves seeking the assistance of a mental health professional. Some of the reasons include financial issues, a change in feelings, a last-ditch effort to see if the relationship can be saved, disagreements over parenting, substance abuse, addictive behaviors (pornography, gambling, video games), lack of trust, emotional or physical abuse, lack of meaningful/ quality time with one another, conflicting values and morals, lack of intimacy or sex, insecurity or self-esteem issues, one person feels as if they are doing more than the other in the relationship, mental health/emotional issues, lack of appreciation or feeling valued, interference from family or friends, stressful jobs, stress in general, lack of compatibility, or they may have simply gotten together for the wrong reasons (feel free to define and imagine an array of possibilities here).

Couples therapy is not limited to those who are experiencing relational difficulties. There are also those couples who, to their credit, are looking for a therapist to help prepare them for marriage by participating in premarital counseling. For many couples, this can prove to be very beneficial, if not necessary. When a couple seeks premarital counseling, there are different ways this can take shape. For some, premarital counseling takes place with the assistance of a licensed mental health professional; others, because of their religious beliefs, may meet with a minister, pastor, or some other type of clergy. Although both types of premarital counseling can be beneficial, there are definitely differences between the two. An individual conducting premarital counseling in a church setting will likely incorporate the couple's faith and religious beliefs. However, a licensed marriage and family therapist will tend to focus on trying to prepare the couple for the realities of married life by addressing challenges they may be currently experiencing or those that may be potential problems.

As a part of the eight-week premarital program I offer my clients, I am very intentional about discussing and examining topics such as their thoughts about what it means to be married and their expectations for the marriage and for one another. We also look at possible financial concerns, unhealthy communication patterns, intimacy, and children (including raising them, parenting styles, and blended families). It's my goal to improve the likelihood of a long, happy, and successful marriage while also increasing their overall understanding of one another. I want to help them have a firm grasp of what it means for them to be married.

I'm sure a lot of clinicians can identify a variety of reasons why couples come to them for help with their relationship. I find it's often due to one of three reasons, or a combination of these. I'll soon go further in depth with each one of these, but for now they are as follows:

- **Communication:** This is a serious challenge with effectively communicating with one another.
- **Infidelity:** More commonly referred to as "cheating," this can be a partner who has literally slept with or emotionally connected with someone who isn't their partner.
- **Expectations:** Often one or both have come to realize that their expectations for the relationship or for the other person are not being met.

CONDUCTING THE COUPLES THERAPY SESSION

When two people come to me seeking help with their relationship, I have several initial objectives. First, I find out what brought them in to see me in the first place. I try to spend an equal amount of time hearing from each in order to learn about their individual perspectives on what the challenges have been. I also pay close attention to more subtle cues, such as how they communicate with one another, how they disagree with each other, and the nonverbal ways in which they interact. I even pay attention to how close they sit to each other. Are their bodies touching? Is there distance between them? If so, how much? What is their individual body language telling me? During this first session, I also learn about each person individually. This may include their history, their family dynamics, their job, and other possible life stressors they may be dealing with. I like to know how they met, what their dating life is like now, or what it used to be. Was their relationship ever on solid ground? If so, what did that look like?

After gaining a sufficient amount of information during that first fifty-minute session, I share my initial observations, describe how I conduct couples therapy sessions, and explain my expectations for them. I inform them that I will likely use a variety of interventions to assist with achieving the desired goals to improve the relationship. Typically, I'll explore whether they have any particular religious or faith-based beliefs, and if they do, I'll likely incorporate that into treatment as well. I also make sure they are aware that I will not be working harder than they will be in therapy. I make it clear that I not only will challenge them during the sessions but also may challenge them outside of the sessions. These challenges may include participating in various activities and exercises or adopting different behaviors toward or ways of thinking about a particular situation or the other person. If they're okay with what they've heard and are willing to adhere to all of this, I let them know that from this point forward we're a team working together to repair and improve the relationship. It's not uncommon for me to thank them for allowing me to be a part of their journey because I know how difficult it can be to open up and share deep and intimate issues with someone they just met.

Unfortunately, from time to time I sit down with a couple and they are not on the same page about much of anything. These individuals will argue, criticize, and blatantly blame the other person (for whatever the issues are) during the first session, and often beyond. In situations like this, I believe that one (or both) simply wants me to "fix" the other person because, apparently, they are the reason the relationship is the way it is. Now, I'm not saying one person's actions can't be the primary reason why there are problems, but exclusively pointing a finger at the other rarely brings about solutions.

I also have to consider the possible impacts that past traumas, addictions, family conflicts, infidelity, or other mental health issues may have on the relationship. In cases like this, individual therapy may be as important as couples therapy, if not more. As a result, I may recommend individual treatment to address personal issues that may be contributing to the problems in the relationship.

During that first meeting, I tend to find myself evaluating how committed each person is to making things better. Every once in a while, I encounter a couple where one of the two already has one foot out of the relationship. These individuals may only be present so they can tell their friends and family (and perhaps even convince themselves) that "I tried everything to save this relationship." In cases like this, the primary purpose of speaking with a counselor becomes reducing feelings of guilt or possible judgment from others.

Now let's take a deeper dive into the three areas I identified earlier where my clients tend to struggle, resulting in them seeking couples therapy.

COMMUNICATION CHALLENGES

All negative emotions, especially anger, depend
for their very existence on your ability to
blame someone or something else for some-
thing in your life that you are not happy about.

—Brian Tracy

I have had so many couples in my office where one agrees that communication problems are significantly and negatively impacting their relationship. So what do communication challenges tend to look like? In my experience, clients say things like "We can't seem to resolve our differences of opinion without it escalating to an argument." Sometimes one person feels like they are misunderstood or not heard, no matter how hard they've tried. On more than one occasion, it has been apparent to me that these two individuals might as well be speaking two different languages. Perhaps one or both are making critical or judgmental remarks to the other. Maybe the tone or even the volume that one or the other uses is triggering their partner. Words can be hurtful and lead to their partner feeling insulted and disrespected. When there is a strong disagreement or difficulty understanding one another's opinions, things can become intense. What does intensity look like? It's just what you think it is: yelling, name-calling, and using profanity—all of which can be considered emotional abuse. Unfortunately, things may get so out of hand that physical altercations or outright physical abuse occurs.

If you or someone you know is dealing with domestic violence, please consider seeking help. The National Domestic Violence Hotline has trained individuals who are available twenty-four hours a day, seven days a week in order to provide free and confidential support or tools for those in abuse situations. The number is 1-800-799-SAFE (7233).

When a couple communicates in a toxic manner, they tend to develop negative habits or patterns of interaction. Once this occurs, their harmful way of speaking to one another becomes even more common. This then increases the number of arguments, conflicts, and expressions of anger, which ultimately lead to anxiety, emotional pain, hurt feelings, and possible depression. The result? Bigger and bigger wedges develop between the two, damaging their relationship, possibly irreparably.

Even when an argument has stopped, there can be lingering aftereffects. Clients have acknowledged the uneasiness or discomfort that seems to hang in the air after a big dispute. They may purposefully avoid one another, going days or even weeks without speaking. I am often taken aback when a couple sits in my office and begins the session by sharing that this is the first time they've spoken to one another in days, despite living in the same household and possibly even having children.

Now let's look at some specific barriers to productive communication within a relationship.

Anger

Most of us get angry at some point because of a situation or a person. It's hard to imagine two people being in a close, intimate relationship and never becoming upset with one another. We all grew up with different triggers or buttons that can be pushed, causing us to react in ways that are less than flattering. However, far too many times I've seen couples in my office become so mad that they completely lose control of their emotions and words. I have yet to see how raising one's voice or using profanity improves a situation, helps with gaining clarity, or resolves a conflict. If one can't share their perspective and their feelings calmly, it's not likely the problem will be solved. Who wants to be yelled at, disrespected, or belittled, especially by a person who is supposed to love you? When we allow our frustrations and anger to take over, we run the risk of damaging not only the relationship but also the other person and ourselves. Once harmful words fly out of our mouths, there is no way to take them back and no way to know, in the moment, what seeds got planted, or how deeply we may have hurt the other person. When we speak to our partners in very explosive, angry ways, no one wins. It is extremely important to try to communicate your concerns with respect and, if at all possible, with some degree of love. Otherwise, you may only be wounding the spirit of the other person. This inability to effectively manage our anger can also cross over into other relationships, negatively impacting how we speak to our family members, coworkers, neighbors, and friends.

In one session, a person became so upset that they cursed at their partner, stood up, and menacingly postured over them, all the while yelling uncontrollably. There have been instances where one partner became so angry that they walked out. Thank goodness this has only happened a few times, and when it did, the individual who left was able to calm down and return to the session.

Clearly, the words you express in anger, especially toward someone you love, can cause them to experience emotional or mental pain. In many ways, anger is like a razor blade. The tighter you hold the blade, the more damage you do to yourself. Ultimately, the damage will need to be treated; if not, you run the risk of infection and long-term problems that will affect more than just you. These wounds that you inflicted on yourself or the other person will ultimately need to be treated and given time to heal. The longer you hold on to your anger, the more you're hurting yourself, preventing you from experiencing inner peace.

Anger in relationships is often due to someone's needs or desires being unmet. If you're reading this and you or someone you know struggles with managing their anger, please consider this: Hurt people tend to hurt people. Broken people tend to break people. So if you or someone you love frequently lashes out in anger, there is some internal work and healing that needs to be done. Perhaps it was their upbringing; maybe past traumas or experiences are playing a role. Maybe there are some mental or physical health issues behind their tendency to lash out. A therapist can often help with examining these factors, working through them, and ideally providing a way for healing to take place. There are also plenty of books, programs, YouTube videos, and podcasts that address anger management that may help a person struggling with this issue. If one is spiritual or religious, praying is not a bad idea either.

Difficulties Listening and Understanding

Hopefully you agree that effective communication is a two-way street. This means two people are able to share their perspectives but also, and perhaps more importantly, able to listen and try to understand the other person's point of view. This can be difficult, especially in the midst of a heated argument. However, it's necessary if a couple hopes to resolve the issue. In couples therapy sessions, there have been times when I've had to serve as somewhat of a referee, directing or encouraging each person to wait until the other has finished their thought before responding, interrupting, or contradicting what is being said. I then have to assess if what one individual stated was heard and understood by the other. If it was not, I step in and try to reframe what was said to provide some clarity to what the other is trying to express.

On occasion, one of the tools I've used is the principles behind Gary Chapman's book *The 5 Love Languages*. These principles can sometimes assist a couple to better understand one another. In case you are unfamiliar with this author and his many books, he created a guide to help people improve their connections with one another by becoming more aware of how they love or feel when they are being loved.[1] It is a useful tool to discover what your significant other desires most in the relationship. In addition, there is plenty of information online about this material, including quizzes to help you determine your love language and your partner's as well.

Being able to listen and understand an individual is a matter of wanting to learn what I call "the emotional support language" of the other person. This is demonstrated when an individual expresses their emotional needs in a way that increases the likelihood of that need being met. I've had sessions where it feels as if the two people sitting before me are speaking totally different languages and become increasingly frustrated with each other. They appear unable to understand the points each is trying to make.

Another way to create healthy communication patterns is to try to avoid repeating your point (or frustrations). No matter what type of relationship it is, people can get tired of being told the same thing over and over again. Making one's point repetitively, hour after hour, day after day, doesn't solve the issue. As a matter of fact, it increases the likelihood of making the other person annoyed, frustrated, or angry. The person you're venting to might even become numb to the problem and then shut down. Once that occurs, you're now doing nothing more than wasting your time and theirs.

In many ways, repeating a point is similar to hammering a nail into a piece of wood. At some point, the nail is not going any deeper. Hammering on the same spot will likely begin to damage the wood (maybe even the nail as well). If a person really doesn't feel like they're being heard, perhaps they should try to find other ways to get the message across. They could consider communicating their concerns at a different time, on a different day, when the other person is in a better mood, or try using the assistance of a therapist (or another neutral third party) to get their opinion heard and understood.

The Need to Be Right

*The key to communication is not what we say,
but rather the attitude that lies behind what
we say.*

—Marianne Williamson

We live in a world where, thanks to social media platforms, everyone can share their opinions with any and everyone. This has led many to believe that whatever they have to tell the world, they're right. In today's society, opinions have become facts. So much so that nowadays, if a person makes a strong point that is shared by another, someone may actually respond out loud and say, "Facts!" I'm not sure how we got here, but we now seem to have a world full of know-it-alls. This has also made us increasingly unwilling to listen to or try to understand someone else's perspective, even though their opinion may have some validity and be just as valuable.

I strongly believe that very few issues are black and white. Life is typically more complicated than we'd like it to be. There's far more to our existence, far more to individuals, far more to situations, and far more to our world than what we see or can truly know. I've often said to friends, family, and clients that there is significantly more that we *don't* know and less of what we *do* know. We live in a world of color, diversity, and a wide-ranging spectrum of possibilities with everything and everyone. There are very few, if any, absolutes, but that doesn't appear to be how many of us see things today. In my opinion, when someone acts as if they have all the answers, that's a demonstration of arrogance, possibly even bordering on narcissism. The people who are the wisest are those who know that they *don't* know everything and are therefore open to learning something new. This is one way toward personal growth.

Unfortunately, this strong desire to be right is often very prevalent in couples and makes it difficult to resolve their issues in therapy. In many types of relationships (friendships, work relationships, family), and especially with couples, people feel strongly that whatever it is they think, feel, or believe is right and unquestionable. Of course, you can see how two people with different points of view, who believe what they're saying is factual, could have a heated argument.

To assist couples where one is confident that they are right and the other is therefore wrong, I share with them what I call the "picture-taking metaphor." During a session, a couple is typically sitting on the couch, and I'm in a single chair anywhere from four to six feet away. I then ask them, if they both pulled out their cell phones and took my picture, would the images be exactly the same? They always respond with a no. I then ask, "Why not?" They are quick to understand that it's not possible because they are not sitting in the exact same spot; therefore, their images can't be identical. They each are taking a picture from a different perspective. This means neither image is wrong, so they both are right. This can also be true when a couple is having a disagreement. There are times when neither is actually wrong; they're just looking at the issue from a different angle or through the lens of their own life experiences. And there may be things that can be learned from the other's point of view.

Me and my ego like being right just as much as the next person. However, in my early twenties (when I thought I was right about everything), I learned something from watching *The Oprah Winfrey Show* that I still carry with me to this day. It was during a time when Oprah had a syndicated program that aired in Chicago at 9:00 a.m. The TV had been on, but I was busy moving about the house, not paying much attention, while preparing to leave for work. I don't know what the topic was or who the guest was for that day, but at some point before I turned the television off, she turned to the audience, as well as to the viewers at home, and made a statement, one she apparently had said many times: "Do I want to be right, or do I want peace?"[2] I stood there, practically overwhelmed as I began to realize how much wisdom was in that question.

From that point on, I put more consideration into whether I needed to invest a lot of time and energy into proving I was right (about whatever the topic was) and, therefore, they were wrong. When disagreements came up with friends, family, or girlfriends, I would simply ask myself, "Is being right worth losing my inner peace at this moment?" Now, don't get me wrong, there were times I felt the need to take a stand in order to get my point across. However, there were many more times when arguing really wasn't necessary and definitely not worth jeopardizing my peace. Usually, after a heated debate, even if I made the stronger argument and *won* the dispute (in my mind), the other person was left in a bad mood, creating distance between us.

Tone of Voice and Delivery

There was a period in my marriage when I was saying things that, unknowingly, negatively impacted my wife. I had a tendency to ask questions about why she chose to do, or not do, certain things around the house. Sometimes I would ask why she would choose to do something in a particular way or at a particular time. This became triggering for her; in other words, this would often annoy her and make her mad. How often I did this, combined with my *tone of voice*, made it come across as criticism. I promise you that was never my intention. My wife is my best friend, and for most of us, we would never purposefully hurt our best friend. Unfortunately, once she was upset, she wouldn't hesitate to let me know that if I had issues with how something was being done, then perhaps I should do it myself. After many attempts to resolve this communication issue, it became apparent what was taking place. You see, I've always been a very curious person. Even as a young child, I frequently asked questions. A lot of questions! I was one of those kids whom you would tell something to, and I would say, "But why?" I wasn't intentionally being disrespectful; I simply wanted to understand something. And that remains true for me even to this day. But I now realized that my curiosity was coming across as criticism about how she was doing things in our home or in our marriage. These days, I'm conscious of when and how I ask my wife questions. I try to make my inquiries in a loving, supportive way without a critical, judgmental tone. To assist with this, I now preface my questions with statements such as "I'm just curious" or "That's interesting. Tell me more . . ." I'll use phrases or a tone of voice that makes it clear I am in no way communicating she is doing something wrong.

Infidelity

As you can probably imagine, many couples come to therapy because of infidelity. At least a third of my clients are trying to deal with a situation where one, and occasionally both, have been unfaithful. "Some national surveys indicate that 15 percent of women and 25 percent of men have experienced intercourse outside of their long-term relationship."[3] I define infidelity as one or both parties having gone outside of an agreed-upon, committed relationship or marriage in order to be intimate with another person. Of course, this could mean having sex with another person, but sometimes what I call "emotional cheating" (which I'll discuss in more detail later) occurs as well.

Intimacy Outside of the Relationship

I do not condone nor am I a believer in extramarital affairs. Having said that, I also think people are free to choose the lifestyle they want to lead, especially if the couple agrees to have what's referred to as an open relationship, or be "swingers." When individuals go outside of their committed relationship in secret, their partners experience disappointment, a loss of trust, and emotional pain. Whether you believe it's justifiable or not, there are a variety of reasons why an individual may choose to step outside their relationship and become involved with another person, which may or may not include being physically intimate or having sex.

The following are some of the reasons why someone would or may cheat:

- They want to escape from the tension or frequent conflicts of their primary relationship.
- The *other* woman/man makes them feel important, understood, special, or needed, feeding their ego.
- There is a lack of emotional connection.
- They are no longer physically attracted to their partner (if they ever were).
- Seeking the excitement or the variety of being with another person sexually appears thrilling.
- The person has a history of cheating.
- Boredom has set in, dulling their current relationship.
- The person has a history of commitment issues.

- One partner is struggling with addiction (drugs, alcohol, sex, pornography, etc.).
- The person has a lack of self-discipline or self-restraint.
- They feel they are entitled to cheat.
- They believe monogamy is not desirable or natural.
- They grew up in a home where infidelity was present or normalized.
- One or both people have psychological or mental health issues.
- One partner is seeking payback because their significant other cheated in the past.
- There are multiple opportunities to be with other people.
- One or both people experienced trauma as an adult or as a child.
- Their feelings for their partner have waned.

Emotional Cheating

A person in a committed relationship is emotional cheating when they are experiencing a very close connection with another person, and therefore, as a part of this connection, they are doing or sharing things that they should probably be doing or sharing with their partner, even if there is no sex (or sexual acts) taking place at all. Examples include sharing deep, personal secrets (including struggles that they are experiencing in their committed relationship), and spending a significant amount of time communicating with, traveling with, enjoying time with, or spending money on the other person instead of their partner.

It's very beneficial, if not necessary, that relationships have clearly defined boundaries and expectations. Hopefully, this will prevent certain lines from being crossed that could cause problems for everyone involved. It is fine to have friends whom you talk to or share things with (regardless of their sex). However, if that relationship is unknown to your partner, that's a sign that this could be emotional cheating. This is especially true if it ultimately negatively impacts the primary relationship.

WORKING WITH COUPLES DEALING WITH INFIDELITY

When a couple shares that they are seeking counseling due to one or both cheating, I immediately realize two things: One, someone is hurting. Two, the trust between them has been violated. The emotional pain caused by infidelity can be very difficult to deal with. The situation can be so upsetting for clients that it is likely to cause depression, anxiety, stress, and possibly even physical ailments. I have yet to find a way to help someone quickly heal after their partner has been intimately involved with someone else. I would love to microwave the process of healing and forgiving, but some things take time to cook. How much and how long will it take? That's a tough question to answer and depends on the individuals and a host of other factors, including how sincere they are about overcoming their situation. Unfortunately, the trust never returns for some. When that happens, people either stay together and never truly feel emotionally safe, or decide they can't live like this and walk away from the relationship.

I have found that, of the men who step outside of the relationship, there are those who truly feel remorseful and those who are not. The latter seem to prefer to minimize their deeds. With men like this, I hear things like, "Yeah, I cheated, but that was then." Or "That was a long time ago!" Or "Why can't she move on? She keeps bringing it up. I said I'm sorry multiple times." Some men even blame their partners for their involvement with other women. In this case, they say things like, "Well, if she would have . . ." Or "If she didn't . . ." In these situations, the man is not taking full responsibility for his actions while also minimizing the feelings of his partner. However, I understand the man's frustrations if he truly wants to move forward but struggles to know how. There are times when a partner seems stuck and becomes emotionally and physically distant. The woman (or other person) may, purposefully or not, say or do things to punish the other for their transgression instead of truly trying to heal and grow. (And I definitely understand why they may behave this way.) When infidelity occurs between people who truly love each other, the pain runs deep. Both parties have a lot to think about and must realize that it takes time to heal emotional wounds, just like physical ones.

It's really unfortunate and challenging for me as a therapist to hear a couple admit that there is no trust in the relationship. They don't trust what they do, where they go, or who they converse with. Quite a few clients have checked their partner's emails, text messages, social media accounts, and cell phone locations; physically followed their partner; or hired a private investigator. They don't trust them to maintain appropriate boundaries with others for fear that a romantic or sexual relationship may occur. They may not trust them with their friends and their coworkers. And they'll definitely be suspicious if their significant other is late getting home, not answering their cell phone, or not responding to text messages. These are just a few of the consequences that can occur when one individual truly doesn't trust the other.

Rebuilding Confidence and Faith

Reestablishing trust is a key component of moving forward when a couple is trying to overcome infidelity. Trust is necessary for any relationship where there is a strong connection. When trying to rebuild trust after infidelity, there are three questions that are important to consider. First, what should the cheating partner try to do? Second, what should the person who was cheated on try to do? And third, what goals should they focus on as a couple?

Now let's take a closer look at each of these.

What Should the Cheating Partner Do After Infidelity?

- Take ownership of and responsibility for what they did, which also means sincerely apologizing. (This likely will happen more than a few times, and this may be necessary.)
- Ask and learn what the other person may need (to help with healing) at this moment, on this day, this week, this month, and this year.
- Do whatever it takes to help their partner feel like they matter, are important, are seen, are heard, are appreciated, and are loved.
- Be honest and transparent. Their words must match their actions, and their actions should align with their words.
- Try their best to validate and understand their partner's feelings. No one wants their thoughts or emotions ignored, dismissed, or minimized.
- Terminate the *other* relationship.
- Work on and better understand themselves, their past, their thoughts and feelings, and why they

cheated. This will hopefully prevent it from occurring again.

What Should the Cheated-On Partner Do After Infidelity?

• Take time to work on healing themselves. This
  could mean a variety of things: going to individual therapy; utilizing materials/books that
  promote recovering from infidelity; investing
  time in self-care activities, especially those that
  nurture the mind; and taking care of their body
  and feeding their spirit. (Many of these things will
  be discussed in greater detail in the chapter on
  self-care.)

• Be honest with themselves and their feelings.

• Consider joining a support group or finding others who are in or have had similar experiences.

• Lean on the support of good friends and family
  (i.e., people who can support them by being a
  good listener and not being judgmental, negative,
  or critical by saying, for example, "I knew they
  weren't right for you all along," or "I hope you
  learned your lesson.")

• Avoid blaming or beating themselves up for what
  has transpired.

• Be patient with themselves and their healing/
  recovery.

• If they have a particular faith or religious belief,
  then pray (for their healing, for their partner, and
  for the relationship).

• Know and believe that they are worthy of receiving respect, honesty, loyalty, and love.

• Show and express love for themselves.

What Should Couples Do After Infidelity?

- If it is possible and agreed on, do as many things together as they can; create new and positive experiences. This includes eating together, traveling together, playing together, and praying together (if your belief system allows).
- Attempt to strengthen the friendship and the foundation of the relationship by talking and listening more to one another (regardless of how uncomfortable the discussions may be).
- Accept and acknowledge that to *grow* through this, it will take time and require patience from each of you.
- Locate a good clinician and do couples therapy.

EXPECTATIONS

Many issues that we encounter in our relationships—whether they be romantic or not, and whether they are with coworkers, friends, or even our family members—are often the result of our expectations. We all hope that people will behave in certain ways and that these behaviors will match what we ultimately want. Parents expect children to obey and get good grades. Close friends expect one another to be there when they go through a difficult time. Most of us expect to be treated appropriately and fairly by our employers. We expect good customer service when we go shopping or out to eat (or at least expect our food order to be correct!). Although we all have expectations that we place on many people, it is often the unmet expectations of those we love, or are in an intimate relationship with, that can cause us to experience the most disappointment, frustration, and pain.

WHAT DO WE EXPECT IN AN
INTIMATE RELATIONSHIP?

When it comes to relationships, there are so many things we feel should be present. Some expect their significant other to love them a certain way, to talk to them a certain way, to listen a certain way, to be interested in what they're interested in, to see things the way they see them, and to share the same morals, values, or beliefs. Some expectations may be considered reasonable or normal, such as the desire to get married, the belief their spouse will be faithful and loyal, that there will be respect in the relationship, and that the couple will spend quality time together. Other expectations are excessive or unrealistic for some, exemplified by statements such as "You're not allowed to have friends of the opposite sex," "You'll have to change your religion," "Obey me at all times," "We'll always have great sex," "This relationship will cure all my personal problems," "You'll have to change your diet and eat what I eat," "We will never have a disagreement," "You will need to change how you dress," "When we have sex, certain things must occur," and "I always know what you're thinking." Whether the expectations are extreme or more typical, we all have them for our partners. But in an intimate connection, unmet expectations may jeopardize the relationship and its future, making therapy something to consider.

I believe each of us is guilty of having a picture in our head of how we want our loved one to treat us and to love us. We also have an image of how we want the overall relationship to look. This can be influenced by several factors, including how we think others will view our relationship. I've seen individuals in therapy cling so tightly to whatever picture they have in their mind that when things turn out differently than they expected, they're simply overcome with disappointment or anger. They may be angry at their situation, the other person, how the other responded, or how they didn't respond. People sometimes feel there must be a particular outcome; otherwise, the hell with it. It's the typical "it's my way or the highway" attitude.

When something isn't going the way we would like it to, or our reality isn't lining up with the image in our head, we should pause and think before we overreact and make matters worse. When someone's actions don't match the ideal we have created, it doesn't mean the picture is necessarily wrong. If we can avoid being narrow-minded, we may gain a greater understanding, which leads to increased insight. Perhaps we'll come to realize that, just because the vision doesn't match what we think it should be, it doesn't necessarily mean this other outcome might not be beneficial or better.

For some of us, our strong, demanding desires and expectations are us basically being selfish. Of course, we're all selfish from time to time, often justifiably so. But when I'm conducting a couples therapy session, individuals can become so focused on things being a certain way (their way) that it can come off to the other person as controlling. Once one person feels that the other is trying to dictate what happens in the relationship, there tends to be resistance, resulting in arguments or disagreements. This is especially true if each party decides to stand their ground and refuse to allow their opinion to be swayed. This is where I attempt to help them understand that the other person has concerns that are legitimate or, at the very least, worth listening to and considering. I also try to help them find common ground and remind them of the love and appreciation they have for one another, with the ultimate goal of preventing the relationship from becoming damaged, distant, or difficult.

Unmet Expectations and the Toxic Environment

No matter what the issue is, no matter what the difference of opinion is, no matter what one's expectation is for the other, no one wants to come home to a house filled with anger, stress, and tension. I've had multiple clients who try to find any excuse to stay away from their home, demonstrated by putting in long hours at work, running errands before arriving home, going to a bar, spending time with friends, or putting in too many hours at the gym (and perhaps not even working out while there).

Many people know how frustrating it can feel to not be comfortable in your own home, avoiding conversation with your partner for fear one comment will quickly escalate into a full-blown argument. This is often referred to as "walking on eggshells." Who benefits from that? No one! Not the couple and not the kids (if there are any present). I don't even think a dog would want to live in a toxic home filled with constant arguing.

I remember not too long ago, my wife and I got into a discussion—not necessarily an argument—in which her words made me feel like I was being attacked. This, in turn, made me defensive and caused me to *express myself*. Afterward, my insides—or better said, my *spirit*—felt uncomfortable, uneasy, and disturbed. I am confident that she felt the same. I didn't like the uncomfortable energy that was present as a result. It simply didn't feel good. I ended up spending a significant amount of time thinking about what took place. I asked myself, "What can I learn from this disagreement? What can I do to prevent this situation from occurring again?" One of the things I realized was that when I'm trying to communicate with my wife, I should strive to honor the individuality we each possess and to communicate, to the best of my ability, with love and respect. After all, we are two different people on two different life journeys. What feels like my personal truth is just that—mine. She has hers too. If you are able to do this consistently, understanding one another will likely increase. Disagreements can then be reduced and will be less intense.

OTHER CHALLENGES THAT CAN NEGATIVELY IMPACT A RELATIONSHIP

As mentioned at the beginning of this chapter, there is a wide variety of issues that may produce challenges in a relationship. Up until this point, I've cited the most common ones I've encountered when providing couples therapy. Now let's look at some others that can also be problematic.

Little to No Intimacy

Intimacy is extremely important and necessary for maintaining a relationship and helping it grow and evolve. Looking at the subheading above, you may be thinking I'm referring to little to no *sex*. And yes, I am; however, *at this moment* I'm also referring to the emotional closeness between two people that conveys warmth, familiarity, and friendship. As human beings, we innately want that special connection with someone who makes us feel desired, valued, appreciated, and loved. Who doesn't want that?

You can often observe the intimacy level between two people by how well they communicate verbally (by the words they use as well as by their tone of voice) and nonverbally (through body language and physical closeness). When a couple has a healthy and positive connection, they can feel at ease even when neither is speaking. These individuals take the time to understand the other's feelings, thoughts, and actions (or at least they try to, to the best of their ability). When intimacy is present, they accept one another unconditionally for who they truly are. Intimacy can also be demonstrated by how much they enjoy being in each other's company, no matter what it is they're doing. Whether they're going out to dinner, picking up items at the grocery store, or simply watching TV, some couples appear to naturally display a strong connection with one another.

I've seen couples who lack intimacy, and I couldn't help but wonder how much longer their relationship will survive. When a person believes intimacy is nonexistent, they will often feel insecure, causing a variety of thoughts to cross their minds. For example, they may wonder, *Is she still interested in me? Is he cheating? Is she no longer physically attracted to me? How come we don't do the things we used to do? Why don't we talk to one another the way we once did?* Individuals raising these questions typically no longer feel safe in the relationship. And for most of us, once we start raising these questions, our imaginations will start trying to provide answers that may or may not be true. It's also not uncommon that when intimacy is lacking, some may, unfortunately, seek comfort or connection outside of their current relationship. Once this occurs, the relationship is further damaged, making it even more difficult to repair and increasing the likelihood of the relationship ending.

The Sexless Relationship

Okay, let's talk about sex (or in this case, the lack thereof). Over the years of being a licensed marriage and family therapist, I have been quite surprised to learn how many couples—who are physically healthy and not considered elderly—go extended periods of time with limited or no sexual intercourse. I have had clients disclose that they haven't had sex with their partner in weeks or months. Some have only engaged in sex once or twice that year, typically on special occasions like birthdays, anniversaries, or holidays.

Now, there are, of course, a variety of reasons I've seen for this. For example, one person, often the male, simply has lost his sexual drive, perhaps due to a medical issue (e.g., poor diet, low testosterone, lack of exercise, stress, poor sleep, age, chronic illness, pain, anxiety, depression). I've seen instances where the male may be experiencing erectile difficulty, possibly struggling with getting or staying aroused. As a result of this issue, the male may become stressed or anxious and therefore put pressure on himself to perform. The partner may unknowingly be adding stress to the situation by making comments such as "What's wrong with you?" Or "Is that it?"

Sometimes males aren't aware of it, but pornography can also negatively impact a couple's ability to have sex. Men have admitted to me that they watch a lot of porn. You may ask, "What is 'a lot' of porn?" I don't have a definitive answer, but what I will say is that *addiction* is when someone is engaged in behaviors that are so self-consuming, they negatively impact one's ability to function in their daily life, leading to problems in their relationships and maybe even their job performance. Pornography is a secretive addiction that needs further attention and study, especially since it is so accessible to everyone, including children and teenagers.

It is not uncommon that those addicted to porn require more specific and sometimes unique sexual encounters in order to become aroused and/or climax. In many ways, it's similar to other addictions, where your body and brain become accustomed to the previous amount of pleasure or stimuli and, over time, crave even more. This is not my area of expertise; however, there is plenty of detailed information out there, including books and videos, regarding addiction. Couples experiencing any of the above challenges may also want to consider seeking professional help from a sex therapist or someone qualified to help individuals and couples with these challenges.

Men aren't the only ones who struggle in the area of sexual intercourse. Women can also have a physiological or psychological problem, causing them to no longer desire sex or to have difficulty engaging in sex. Women may be diagnosed with female orgasmic disorder, female sexual interest/arousal disorder, or genito-pelvic pain/penetration disorder. I won't get into defining each of these, since that is not the primary focus of this book; however, speak to a licensed professional or a doctor, visit your public library, or go online, and I'm sure you will find very detailed information about these conditions. A woman's past sexual experiences or trauma could also cause her to be reluctant to have or disinterested in having sex. Something as simple as frequent arguments or lack of support in the home can cause a woman to lose interest in, or affect their desire to have sex with, their partner.

Now let's look at some other reasons for a sexless relationship. It's possible that one person is withholding sex as a way of punishing the other, using sex as a weapon. For example, a person may decide that because their partner *didn't* do something, or the person *did* do something that was unacceptable, there will be no sex. Perhaps one person has been emotionally or mentally hurt recently, thus it becomes tough for them to "be in the mood," especially if even being in the same bed doesn't feel comfortable, desirable, or safe.

Unfortunately, there have been a few instances in my sessions when the male in a heterosexual relationship has expressed his belief that regardless of whether his partner is in the mood or not, it is her duty to sexually satisfy him. I don't agree with this attitude; I consider it sexist. However, when I'm dealing with situations like this, it's my job to attempt to first better understand the man's beliefs and where they came from. After gaining that info, hopefully I can find a way to get him to be more open-minded, see things from his partner's perspective, and have some degree of empathy. Of course, I also examine any other issues that are present in the relationship that may cause them to struggle sexually, or sexual compatibility.

Money, Money, Money!

It's been said that "money is the root of all evil." I don't believe that to be true. (However, the *pursuit* of money can definitely produce negative consequences.) But I can say that when two people in a relationship, especially if they live together, don't see eye to eye on the subject of money, there will be a greater likelihood of conflicts and arguments. As I stated before, we all come from different backgrounds and different families. Therefore the value individuals place on money and their spending and saving habits will be different. I've observed relationships where one person is "the spender," while the other tends to be "the saver." There's absolutely nothing wrong with this, and if they're willing to work together, they may actually balance one another out. I recommend that when it comes to household finances and money in general, both parties do their best to understand and respect the thoughts and opinions of their partner. Sometimes, in order to work together, a couple may need to consider ways to compromise, make sacrifices, or do things a little differently than how they would if they were on their own. If two people are finding it difficult to resolve differences of opinion regarding money, a therapist may help. An alternative is sitting down with a financial adviser, who can help address a variety of money-related challenges while also providing a plan for the couple's financial future. At the very least, it may not be a bad idea to simply pick up some books on money and finances and read them together.

Children

Raising children is considered by many to be one of the most challenging as well as one of the most important jobs a person can undertake. When two parents are able to collaborate on raising healthy, happy, ethical, kind, and intelligent children, the world is a better place for their efforts. However, when parents can't seem to agree on what's in the children's best interest, it can create a very divisive household (not to mention negatively impacting the kids).

It's not uncommon for one person to believe that how they were raised (or at least what they are familiar with) is how their children should be raised. These differences in parenting styles can lead to a lot of discussion or disagreement about, for example, what type of school the kids should go to, how they should be disciplined, what extracurricular activities they should be involved in, what type of clothing is appropriate, what foods they should or shouldn't eat, and what religious beliefs they should be taught, if any. These are all things that people tend to have very strong convictions about and also can become what divides a couple and negatively impacts their relationship. Things become even more convoluted if the child has special needs, whether they be psychological issues or physical disabilities. When different viewpoints on child rearing are so obvious, it's important for parents to be open to trying to understand one another's experiences and ideas. Couples should realize that there are times when both parents have valid points. And they should understand that since they both ultimately want what is best for the child, there is more than one way to accomplish this. There are often many paths to reach a given destination.

SOME RELATIONSHIPS ARE NOT RIGHT FOR US

It is extremely important to be aware of how you are being treated in a relationship. If you feel as if you're being disrespected, ignored, neglected, not valued, not appreciated, threatened, manipulated, taken advantage of, or mentally or physically abused, then you should question if it is in your best interest to remain with this person. You should consider whether this individual is unwilling, unable, or incapable of showing empathy or providing you with the type of relationship you desire. Maybe their history, upbringing, traumas, insecurities, ego, or unhealed wounds or "brokenness" makes them incapable of meeting the emotional needs or expectations of others in a relationship. Perhaps it is you with these issues. Either way, it could be that you two just don't work well together. When I was young, my mom often said, "You can't get blood from a turnip." I understand this to mean there are some situations where the outcome you're looking for just isn't going to happen.

It's unfortunate that so many people struggle with mental health or emotional issues, which also can contribute to a person not being right for us. There are those who have an actual diagnosis, but many more have undiagnosed conditions that make it extremely difficult to be in a healthy relationship. Of course, those who have true mental health challenges are still entitled to be in a relationship and experience the joys of having a loving connection with another human being. It just may take more time and effort to find the right match, one in which there is understanding and acceptance of the person's personal struggles.

It's also possible that it may not be the right time for someone to be in a committed relationship. I believe that, in practically every aspect of life, timing is extremely important. Just as there are different seasons in which certain events happen in nature, likely there are also times where we should probably be single. Maybe we're extremely busy. Perhaps we are dealing with a challenging family situation or feeling overwhelmed as a result of financial or physical health issues. There are times where it's just not a priority, and we simply don't want to be seriously involved with anyone. No matter the situation, people need to determine if it's in their best interest to be in a relationship.

I've also learned that sometimes it's beneficial for the

client to focus on themselves before entering into a relationship. By doing so, they can address areas that need to be examined, resolved, or healed. There may be past or recent traumas that have yet to be dealt with. Perhaps it's time to focus on nurturing the mind, body, or spirit going into therapy to face symptoms such as depression or anxiety. Doing these things just may prevent unnecessary past or present baggage from becoming an obstacle to a healthy relationship in the future.

When it comes to the importance of being as healthy as we can be in a relationship, I have shared with clients what I call "the team sports metaphor." Think of a situation where one member of a five-person basketball team is injured. Depending on the severity, the injury will very likely impact the team's ability to be successful. This is why I encourage people to continually work on themselves by healing old wounds and strengthening areas that could be detrimental to a relationship. Much like being in a relationship, if the player who was injured takes the time to heal, the team will be a much stronger unit and therefore have a greater opportunity for success.

LEAVING VERSUS STAYING

There are times when a relationship may not be abusive or have major conflicts, yet it still is not the right one for you. If you aren't sure, look inside yourself and really consider factors, such as whether they are what you're looking for, whether you are what they're looking for, what your expectations are, and whether this is the right time to even be in a relationship. These and similar questions can be discussed with trusted friends, family, and perhaps a licensed therapist. But also consider that some relationships are simply not meant to last forever (despite what is often depicted in films and on TV). Sometimes people come into our lives for a reason or a season.

Maybe they're there to help us grow or to bring certain things to our awareness. And I definitely don't recommend that anyone try to force a relationship or to change someone in order to make them what they want them to be.

Being in a relationship with someone who has mental health challenges can also make a person question if they are able or willing to remain in the relationship. This is especially true if the individual has issues like an addiction or a *personality disorder*. Personality disorders are usually ongoing or long-lasting mental health conditions that can negatively impact the way a person thinks, feels, and behaves in society, which can be problematic in a relationship. You can look up the various personality disorders on the internet, but if you're unsure whether you or your partner has one of these disorders, a mental health professional should make an official diagnosis.

I also encourage individuals who are involved with someone who has a challenging mental health diagnosis to determine if they are equipped to deal with the various issues that will likely be a part of that relationship. If being with them results in somebody being physically abused, their overall emotional well-being becoming compromised, or someone being taken advantage of, I can't recommend remaining in the relationship. However, in certain situations and within certain parameters, I recommend couples get help from licensed clinicians or those trained to assist couples and/or individuals when a person is struggling to deal with their partner's diagnosis.

I've often worked with women, and in a few cases men, who feel a strong sense of obligation to remain in a destructive relationship, and therefore have a tough time leaving, for a variety of reasons:

- They believe they have to stay together for the sake of the children.

- Their religious/spiritual beliefs do not support divorce.
- They are afraid of what other people may think.
- They feel a sense of obligation to their partner ("I have to be there for them.").
- They worry about how they will support themselves financially without a partner.
- They prefer to be in a bad relationship rather than none at all.
- They are in a "trauma bond" (when an individual who is being abused feels connected or bonded to the abuser).
- They are afraid of the uncertainty that comes with not knowing what their life will look like when they are single.

In any relationship, remember to love yourself. Sometimes loving yourself means recognizing when it's time to leave a relationship because of the harm and pain you are experiencing by remaining in it. I realize this is often easier said than done, and there are usually many things to consider before you make such a decision. An important one being, are they showing you love and respect? If you remain in a relationship that is causing mental or emotional pain, are you showing yourself love and respect? To quote a statement I've seen attributed to author Jay Shetty, "You shouldn't drink poison just because you're thirsty." In a relationship, this means doing your best to avoid being in a harmful or destructive situation simply because you are desperate to feel connected to another person. Know that you deserve better. At the very least, know that you deserve to be treated like a human being, with respect and dignity.

Letting go usually requires us to have a certain amount of inner strength, but even if moving on is hard, that doesn't mean we shouldn't do it. I've had clients in relationships who intellectually knew they should leave but remained anyway. I've seen firsthand how hard it was for them to choose what was in their best interest—to end the relationship. In scenarios like this, I encourage individuals not to beat themselves up, to be patient with themselves, to love themselves, and to try to make even the smallest steps toward achieving their ultimate goal—freedom from their toxic situation. No matter how challenging, uncomfortable, and even painful getting out of these dilemmas can be, a person should try. Medicine may taste disgusting going down, but if it makes us feel better in the end, it's usually worth the initial discomfort.

HOW A RELATIONSHIP ENDING AFFECTS THE KIDS

If a relationship is destined to end, it's important to take a moment to understand what the children (if there are any) may be forced to deal with. I find it frustrating when parents who are separated or divorced use their children as pawns, typically when the couple has a contentious relationship that creates a dynamic where the children prefer one parent over the other. The children are told things that may or may not be true (and should remain private between the adults) in an apparent effort to manipulate their beliefs about the other parent. This is not only confusing to children, but it also likely produces inner conflict and anxiety as they struggle with whom they should remain loyal to. Imagine how challenging this could be for a child, especially when they love both parents. I have seen this lead to children becoming depressed, developing anxiety, experiencing difficulties in school, and having issues with other family members and even peers. In situations like these,

I try to help children understand and deal with their feelings and the changes taking place in their home life—over which they have no control.

When parents decide to divorce, there are several recommendations I ask them to consider when it comes to the children. First, the parents should put aside all feelings of anger and resentment they have for one another and ask, "What's in the best interest of our children? What behaviors can we display that will help them deal with this transition?" I suggest parents talk to each child in order to understand what their children are going through and what thoughts or feelings they may be struggling with. Realize that talking negatively about the other parent to the child likely will not be productive. And finally, family therapy—involving everyone—may prove to be useful, in addition to individual therapy for the child.

CAN COUPLES THERAPY REALLY WORK?

Couples therapy has proven to be very beneficial for many, especially those willing to put in the work and think and do things differently than they have in the past. Throughout my years as a licensed clinician, I have worked with many couples from all walks of life who were struggling with a variety of marital or relational challenges. I honestly felt that some couples were not a healthy match for one another, but that did not stop me from doing my best to help them gain a better understanding of their issues, the other person's point of view, themselves, and the relationship itself.

For couples in more toxic situations, there have been times when we were unable to make the necessary progress for long-lasting, positive change. And over the years, I've learned to accept that repairing a relationship is not solely my responsibility, if at all. What I mean is that if individuals ultimately decide to split up and move on, there is absolutely no reason for me to feel bad, guilty, or like I let them down (something that I experienced in my earlier years as a clinician). The couple is responsible for creating positive change, growth, and healing in their relationship. In many ways, I'm like their personal trainer: I'm there to guide and show them how to make changes, but I can't do it for them. Their progress depends on how much work they're willing to put into it. It is not my intention to work harder than the clients at producing change.

Although some of the couples I've worked with did not reach a "happily ever after" ending, I have been able to help the vast majority. I have seen with my own eyes how couples therapy can be beneficial to two individuals who are struggling with overcoming issues that were previously impacting their relationship in negative ways. These couples were often able to heal themselves and repair their connection. Their lives gradually became filled with new hopes, new possibilities, renewed bonds, healthier communication, reignited love, and an improved ability to work together. They may not have become perfect couples that no longer have disagreements; however, they achieved more peace in their home, in their lives, and in their relationship.

HEALTHY RELATIONSHIPS

What are some of the key attributes I've observed in couples that lead to healthier and happier relationships? I keep certain goals in mind for my marriage, as well as for my clients' relationships. I find that when these attributes are present, they can assist with creating a strong foundation that can be built upon. Here is a list of some of the more common traits I've seen healthy couples display that help them experience positive, long-lasting, and wonderful relationships:

- Being really good friends (if not best friends)
- Frequently attempting to better understand one another's points of view
- Communicating in a healthy way (e.g., finding ways to talk that don't include yelling, profanity, name-calling, criticism, or judgment)
- Creating quality time together
- Being willing to work together to accomplish goals
- Laughing, or being able to laugh together
- Praying together
- Sharing or experiencing one another's interests (hobbies or pleasurable activities) at least occasionally
- Engaging in activities together, from the mundane to the more exotic or romantic
- Being willing to work on themselves, individually, for the betterment of the relationship
- Understanding when and what makes their partner feel that they are loved
- Identifying and engaging in *their* agreed-upon ways of experiencing intimacy
- *Going* through things together while understanding the value of *growing* through things together
- Frequently demonstrating and expressing love for one another
- Not taking one another for granted
- Supporting one another through life's challenges (health, career, family)
- Having a healthy respect for one another
- Realizing they are better and happier as individuals because of the health of their relationship

I'm sure there are others I have missed, but I would also

like to stress the importance of having patience. Change, especially positive change, takes time. How much time? Who knows; we are all different with different life experiences, expectations, and mindsets. Many of us struggle with being patient because when we want change, we want it now! We live in the world of microwavable food and the ability to choose people by swiping left or right. However, anything worth truly having is worth working on and waiting for.

No one ever said being in an intimate relationship is easy. Sometimes those struggles may help us grow as individuals as well as a couple, allowing us to learn about each other and experience love at deeper and deeper levels. I believe that if we're with the right person—an individual who is loving, supportive, trusting, and understanding—the quality of our lives can be enhanced significantly while allowing us to feel more joy and even accomplish much more than we could have on our own.

CHAPTER 4

Lessons Learned About Nonromantic Relationships

In every relationship, in every moment, we teach either love or fear.

—Marianne Williamson

September 29, 1998
Burbank, California

> *I wish I knew what is wrong with me. I wish I knew what is wrong with my life. There have been times lately where I'm not even sure why I'm here. Why am I here on this planet? I used to think that I was here for others, you know, my friends and family, maybe in some cases for total strangers. But being in Los Angeles*

*and not really having friends here, my purpose
doesn't seem to be the same.*

What you just read was taken from an old journal of mine when I was living in Southern California. At the time of that writing, I had been living there for about a year after having relocated from Chicago. I had a couple of friends I knew prior to moving to LA, but they were often busy leading their own lives. And I had nothing that even came close to resembling a romantic relationship, let alone a dating life. Looking back, I don't believe *not* being in a relationship was really that big a deal for me. I'm pretty sure my real problem was not only trying to manage being alone as much as I was, but also dealing with what seemed like overwhelming loneliness and a lack of friends I could spend time with.

During that time, I experienced varying degrees of sadness and depression. I remember instances when I would spend entire weekends without talking to a single soul. I would try to reach out to my friends back in Chicago, but so often they didn't answer their phones. I'd leave messages and would eventually get a return call, but most likely it was on another day or perhaps even a week or two later. I don't believe that any of my friends back home were intentionally ignoring me; they were simply dealing with their own stuff. As a result, though, I got to feel firsthand how important our nonromantic relationships are. Having people to share your life with, your personal struggles with, or even laugh with can provide meaning and a sense of connection.

In our society, a lot of importance is placed on intimate relationships. Our friends and family share their stories of meeting people, falling in love, getting married, or even falling out of love and the heartache that follows. There are countless TV shows and movies that promote intimate relationships as a near necessity for all human beings. And social media only increases the focus, as people have a tendency to want to share what they're doing with their partners or promote an image of how they want you to view their romantic relationships.

However, as great as a healthy intimate relationship can be, there are other people who play just as important a role in our lives and our overall sense of well-being. It's these other relationships that I'll discuss in this chapter. I'll look at how we interact with one another, our desires for connection, the expectations we place on those in our lives, and how our egos and insecurities can damage relationships. If we can improve how we interact with one another, the positive impact that we can make in the world would be limitless.

WE'RE ALL ON A JOURNEY

If you haven't already heard this saying (attributed to several people, including Ian Maclaren and Robin Williams), take a moment to consider it: "Everyone you meet is fighting a battle you know nothing about. Be kind. Always."[1]

Everyone (whether they're a client of mine or not) has situations they are going through, obstacles they're trying to overcome, or issues that have been very difficult to manage. Sometimes we don't take the time to realize that that person we may be judging could be dealing with something we would not be able to handle. You don't know me any more than I know you, but we both have our strengths, our weaknesses, and our struggles. As a clinician, I've learned that so many of us are often trying to overcome dysfunctional or toxic experiences from our past, potentially mentally or emotionally damaging experiences that are the result of the families we grew up in.

We have all seen how our relationships with others significantly impact the quality of our lives and our sense of well-being. Hopefully, those currently in our lives provide us the opportunity to experience positive connections, love, affection, and joyful moments. Relationships can also give us opportunities to examine parts of ourselves or our character that we may need to work on to become better individuals. Maybe some people are in our lives for a larger, previously unknown purpose, such as to help us figure out how to be a better spouse, friend, sibling, or coworker. Relationships can also help us see our unhealed wounds or the parts of us that we need to address in order to continue *our journey* of personal growth.

THE IMPORTANCE OF HEALTHY, POSITIVE RELATIONSHIPS

I'll start out by briefly looking at what happens when we *don't* have quality relationships in our lives. Here are two unfortunate facts: According to the National Institute on Aging, loneliness can be so detrimental to our health that it is the equivalent of smoking fifteen cigarettes a day.[2] According to former surgeon general Vivek Murthy, this can result in shortening a person's lifespan by fifteen years.[3]

We are social creatures; therefore the vast majority of us have an innate desire to feel a sense of belonging or connection to others. Our desire to bond is so strong that it's probably one reason why people join social groups like book clubs, churches, athletic/intramural teams, fraternities, sororities, political parties, and even street gangs. It's us wanting to feel that connection with others where we feel safe, supported, seen, heard, and validated, especially by those we share common interests with.

Could it be that a major reason why we have so many problems in our world today is our inability to truly connect with one another? Maybe I'd have fewer clients if people didn't feel so isolated and alone. Perhaps we don't do as good a job as we need to with helping others feel as if they belong.

We are clearly happier when we feel connected to others. Think about any challenging issue in our world today or in your personal life. Wouldn't it be a little easier to deal with if there was someone there by your side to help? Healthy, positive connections promote healing while disconnection promotes pain, or "dis-ease." When we don't have connections, or feel connected, it can affect our ability to accomplish goals, negatively impact our self-esteem/self-worth, hamper our work performance, cause a lack of motivation, and significantly impact both our mental and physical health.

Just as we can see the impact when we're lacking quality relationships, we can also see how we can be impacted positively by quality relationships. Those who have a strong sense of connection with others tend to be happier, laugh more, accomplish more, experience less depression, be better equipped to deal with life's stressors, and even look better. Our relationships can be our greatest teachers. They can also be conduits to both our healing and growth.

Now let's look at the various types of relationships that can impact a client's mental health, the mental health of someone you may know, and maybe yours as well.

OUR FRIENDSHIPS

Having quality friendships can make dealing with life's challenges easier. I have had a countless number of clients who, due to a lack of friendships (or quality friendships), are either often alone, feel lonely, or so focused on taking care of their immediate family that they don't have the time to nurture friendships.

There are many benefits to having quality relationships. Healthy, positive friendships help us to avoid feeling alone or being lonely. We gain not only the opportunity to feel supported but also the chance to support others. In truly meaningful friendships, we can learn about ourselves based on how we respond or interact with others. Some friends help motivate us to do or achieve more; on other occasions, they can support us if we fall short of our goals.

When I use the term "quality friendships," I'm referring to relationships where an individual feels like the other person or people are there for them in any way that's needed. These are relationships where you feel safe, where there is trust, and where you know that they are there to support you no matter what challenge you might be facing. I'm talking about relationships where there is giving and sharing between individuals, where things feel balanced and equal. If one person does all the talking, all the sharing, all the calling, all the reaching out, all the time, then the friendship can become unbalanced. This could result in one person becoming annoyed, questioning the quality of the relationship, or being resentful. In quality friendships, even if things are a little one-sided from time to time, people still accept the other person for who they are— flaws and all.

Of course, everyone gets to define what they consider a "quality friendship." Everyone has their expectations when it comes to healthy connections. But we should be careful with what we expect from another human being. Sometimes what we hope to get from them is something they may not be able to provide. It's very unrealistic to expect a vase that you know has cracks in it to hold water for any substantial amount of time. Nor would I expect someone who grew up in a family that rarely expressed emotions and wasn't physically affectionate to easily make the transition to being part of a family where they are constantly hugging and telling one another how much they love them.

When I reflect on my personal life, I've noticed I have

three types of secure, strong friendships. First, there are those whom I speak with on a regular or semiregular basis. Then there are people whom I talk with perhaps once every two or three months where there is a concerted effort in which we try to remain in touch with one another (these are people who typically don't live in my state). Finally, there are my friends whom I may only speak to once a year or so. But what's great about these relationships is that no matter how much time has elapsed since we last spoke, when we do talk, it feels as if no time has passed at all. It's like we spoke last week and we're picking up where we left off. More than likely you have friendships that fall into these categories. I always ask my clients if they have relationships that they are able to maintain as well. These bonds are what can help people feel emotionally stable and balanced.

Missing or Lacking Friendships

A lack of friendships or close relationships with others can be problematic and become a contributing factor in clients' emotional health challenges. People in this situation either are unsure how to nurture friendships, don't feel they have the time, or have become accustomed to being alone and not spending time with friends. Some may not be fortunate enough to be in an environment where friendships can be easily formed. Unfortunately, when we get older, it appears to become more difficult to establish and develop quality relationships. To solve this problem for myself, I considered joining a fraternity in order to be part of "the brotherhood" and develop the friendships I hoped would follow as a result.

For many men, seeking new friendships is often more difficult since males tend to be more cautious or suspicious when it comes to allowing new guys into their lives. In addition to being slow to trust, most guys I know would be a little reluctant to ask another guy (especially one they recently met) out to get a bite to eat or go see a movie. There are heterosexual men who do not want another man to even remotely question their manhood or gender preference. Yeah, I know it seems ridiculous (and maybe even a little judgmental or homophobic) that some men may feel reluctant or hesitant to ask another to hang out, but that doesn't mean it's not true.

Typically, when I find that a client lacks quality connections with others, I try to explore several things with them. This is especially true if this lack is negatively impacting their mental state or is something they would like to change. I explore with them various areas of their life, including personal interests, to determine if there are groups, activities, clubs, or organizations where they can meet people with similar interests. In these environments, it may be possible to find people to connect with, leading to new and beneficial friendships. I often ask my clients to consider strengthening, repairing, reconnecting, or rebuilding friendships that they already have. It's not a bad idea to reach out to and check in on people from our past whom we've considered our friends but haven't spoken to in a while. Taking the time to let someone know you are thinking about them will be beneficial for the person making the call as well as the one receiving it. Ralph Waldo Emerson said, "The only way to have a friend, is to be a friend."[4] The Bible also chimes in on the subject: "A man who has friends must himself be friendly" (Prov. 18:24 NKJV).

Toxic Friendships

It's weird to put *toxic* in the same sentence with *friendship* because it would seem that if a relationship is in any way unhealthy, let alone damaging, how could that represent friendship? A toxic friendship leads to situations in which an individual feels less-than or gets emotionally hurt as a result of interactions with the other person. These relationships tend to lack trust, may be one-sided, or even cause you to question why you continue talking to them. If, after spending time with a friend or talking to them on the phone, a person feels worse than they did before the interaction, this may be a toxic relationship. Staying in these relationships not only compromises your emotional well-being but also may impact other areas of your life. In our desperation to feel connected to others, sometimes we settle for whatever we feel we can get. But by doing so we could end up in relationships that do us more harm than good.

I have seen instances where one person who is displaying toxic behaviors is unaware that they are frustrating or disappointing another. So many times we are unaware of how our own words, actions, or inactions are negatively impacting someone, even when it's someone we care about. In this case, the person who is upset should try to communicate their feelings, ideally in a loving way that prevents them from becoming defensive. If attempts to smooth things out have proven to be unsuccessful, a person may consider distancing themselves from the toxic friend or, worst-case scenario, ending the relationship altogether.

OUR FAMILY

The relationships we have with our family members are some of the most important and influential relationships we will ever have. They can be extremely fulfilling and loving or produce great frustration and pain.

The topic of family relationships is truly a broad area. Like many of the topics discussed here, it's worthy of its own chapter—or better yet, its own book. Of course, much has been written about families, family struggles, and possible ways to overcome challenges within them. If you'd like to learn more about or better understand family dynamics, I encourage you to explore the information that is available in books, courses, or seminars. Of course, if you have difficult family issues, trauma, or drama present, family therapy should be seriously considered (especially if those involved are open to the idea).

Biological and Surrogate Families

From the moment we're born, our family members are the people with whom we first begin experiencing what it's like to be connected to others. Family is where most of us get our first taste of what it feels like to be loved. Over time, we hopefully begin discovering our own ways to return that love.

The families we're raised in tend to be where the seeds that will impact our lives, our future relationships, and how we interact with others are planted. That's because our families are also where we get exposed to values, morals, and principles (or at least the ones that our family adheres to). We learn what to look for in or expect from others. During this time, when we're young, we're hopefully gaining a variety of important skills that will be of great value as we get older. Some of these skills include (but are not limited to) patience, the value of trust, the importance of being accountable/responsible for our actions, discernment, good decision-making, effective communication, how to resolve differences effectively, empathy/sympathy, the power of forgiveness, kindness, how to nurture relationships, and what it means to be connected to something larger than ourselves. When family members are consistently able to love and support one another "through thick and thin," true growth, happiness, and joy become possible for all.

Unfortunately, in some households there are only a few seeds of positivity planted. In very dysfunctional environments, no positivity is nurtured at all. There are homes where children were never taught, or never saw, loving interactions that demonstrated healthy communication, understanding, and patience. This also tends to be the case for those who are or were responsible for teaching it, were abused, neglected, or never learned it from their family or parents.

The Different Relationships Within a Family

Many relationships can exist within families. Typically, you have the relationship between two parents (clearly not always the case since there are also one-parent households), and then there's the parent's or parents' relationship with the child or children. If there's more than one child, the siblings have their own relationships, as well as those with extended family members, which can include grandparents, aunts, uncles, cousins, nieces, and nephews. Then there's the blended family in which one or both adults bring with them their children from previous relationships; the family now consists of stepchildren and stepparents. Lastly, relationships within a family could include children who've been brought into the home by way of fostering or adoption.

"Family" for a lot of people also includes those to whom we are not related by blood. These are the families that we create ourselves. Our *surrogate family*: the people who always felt like they were family, whom we care deeply for, and who may even have a family title or designation (cousin, brother, sister, dad, uncle, etc.). These may be people who we have known all our lives, grew up with, or feel are just as close as our own biological family. People, including myself, sometimes create surrogate families in order to fill the space that our natural families haven't been able to fill.

I have created a family of my own as a result of the love that I've developed for these people: Uncle Walter and his wife, Auntie Joyce; their late daughter/my cousin, Carla (I miss you, Carla!); my nieces, Kori and Marissa; and my little sister, Kandi, which includes her children, giving me an additional niece and nephew. (I also gained an additional sister during high school. Hi, Phyllis!) These people mean a lot to me, and to varying degrees, they've all played very important roles at different points in my life.

THE DYSFUNCTIONAL-FAMILY SPECTRUM

As a licensed marriage and family therapist, I've learned that many of my clients became my clients because of the families they were raised in. In many ways they are trying to recover from toxic family relationships or experiences that took place while growing up. Some of these family challenges may still exist or have grown progressively worse over time.

Sometimes when we've experienced unhealthy family relationships as children, we may, either knowingly or un- knowingly, reproduce similar problems as adults. Basically, we duplicate or pass down negative behavioral patterns, poten- tially impacting our own offspring. Unfortunately, as import- ant as family is, if our relationships are emotionally damaging, unhealthy, and full of conflict, the pain can be devastating, feel insurmountable, and stay with us throughout our lives.

Working with numerous families, couples, and individuals over the years, I've learned that as much as we all desire an amazing family life that resembles something like *The Brady Bunch* or *The Cosby Show*, that's simply not the reality for most people. After all, those are just television shows created for our entertainment. I remember years ago hearing people blam- ing their struggles on the fact that they were brought up in a "dysfunctional family." But in reality, no family is perfect. We know this logically because no individual person is perfect; therefore, *every* family will have its own challenges.

In many ways, every family has some degree of dysfunction. I have told clients that every family is on what I refer to as "the dysfunctional-family spectrum." This means that to varying degrees, every family has challenges. It comes down to whether they are more on the right side, on the left side, or somewhere in the middle of this scale (where many of us most likely reside). For example, on the left side are families who have issues that are fairly common (but not necessarily easy to deal with), such as divorce, struggles with the loss of a loved one, or challenges with getting all the bills paid on time. Meanwhile, on the right side are families that are forced to deal with issues like hunger and homelessness, and those that repeatedly hurt one another as they struggle with issues like neglect, abuse, addiction, or violence. This level of dysfunction and toxicity often means a significant amount of trauma is also present.

Families will always have disagreements, arguments, or conflicts that their members may find annoying, frustrating, or hurtful. Some of these conflicts create emotional distance between two or more family members, which may start in childhood and extend far into adulthood (unless those involved are willing to try to resolve these issues).

Below is a list of some issues I've seen as a therapist that tend to create toxicity, conflict, division, and emotional distance in families. It's likely that you've seen some of these situations in the lives of people you know; perhaps you've even experienced several of them. If you're a counselor, mediator, life coach, teacher, or family attorney, or you have a job where you help families resolve issues, you will likely recognize some of these challenging family dilemmas:

- Violence and abuse (e.g., sexual abuse, child abuse, elder abuse, physical abuse, emotional abuse, neglect)

- Substance abuse and/or addiction
- Mental health issues (unresolved or unaddressed)
- Addictive behaviors toward pornography or technology/social media (cell phones, video games, social media, TikTok, etc.)
- Children not living up to their parents' expectations (often causing the child to feel pressure or anxiety)
- Parents' divorce
- Disagreements and conflicts due to a teenager's declared or expressed sexual orientation
- Entitled or spoiled young people
- Sibling rivalry
- Unresolved animosity or grudges
- Lack of respect
- Selfishness, regardless of the desires of others
- Disagreements about morals or religious beliefs
- Parents' beliefs that children are not doing assigned tasks, chores, or schoolwork
- Unnecessary criticism or judgment
- Young people who do not obey their parents
- Excessive punishment or consequences placed on the children
- Unrealistic (even delusional) beliefs, hopes, or goals
- Unresolved or unaddressed pain
- Betrayal, disappointment, or abandonment
- Conflicts with the in-laws
- Racist, sexist, or homophobic views that interfere with other family members' outside relationships
- Lack of understanding or being heard
- Parents who had children at a young age or who lack experience
- Absentee or uninvolved parents, or parents who are physically or emotionally distant

- Parents who remain together despite being in a toxic relationship
- Infidelity by one or both parents
- Jealousy and envy
- Financial challenges, including difficulty managing bills, disagreements with how money is spent/saved, and/or stress of being the sole breadwinner
- Overinflated and out-of-control egos
- Refusal to communicate or appropriately discuss issues
- Environmental stressors, such as living in poverty or in a violent neighborhood
- Unfair distribution of responsibilities within the home
- Inability to cope with the death of a beloved family member
- Inability to take responsibility for hurting another family member
- Lying and intentional deception
- Lack of affection or love shown within the home
- Attempts to control or manipulate others
- Discovered family secrets
- Disagreements regarding the raising of the child or children
- The religious or political beliefs of the parents being forced upon the adolescent
- An unwillingness to forgive (depending on the severity of the transgressions)
- Unfair or unjust treatment

Obviously, despite all the items I've listed here, this doesn't encompass every situation that can negatively impact a family.

But these are some of the scenarios I've helped families work through.

Families can be difficult. Everyone may not get along. There will be issues within each home, but that doesn't mean people shouldn't try to resolve ongoing problems. If, however, the challenges cannot be overcome, people are free to make decisions regarding the level of closeness and the type of interactions they want to have with their family members. Hopefully, there will at least be respect between those who have conflicts and that some love will still remain, even if it has to be given at a distance.

OUR RELATIONSHIPS WITH COWORKERS

In most workplaces, we will have coworkers. These are people we work side by side with, including assistants, support staff, supervisors, managers, and owners of the business. Regardless of the role or position an individual is in, the quality of those relationships and interactions can greatly impact the success of the organization, in addition to helping you determine if the workplace environment is healthy or toxic.

Like many people, I have had a variety of positions where the environment was a huge factor in whether I was happy there or not (regardless of how much money I made). For example, I lived in Southern California and worked for *The Howie Mandel Show* for a time. In case you are unfamiliar with Howie, he's a comedian who, among other things, has also been an actor, the voice of Gizmo (from the movie *Gremlins*), a host of various television shows, and is currently (at the time of this writing) a judge on *America's Got Talent*. Now this particular program was a daytime talk show, and my job title was production assistant. This meant I did a variety of things—

basically, whatever the higher-ups told me to do—from picking up lunch to assisting someone in the control room. Sometimes the days were long and the pay was very low. How low? How does five dollars an hour sound? Of course, this was over twenty years ago, but that wasn't great pay even then. However, despite the low salary, I found it to be one of the best places I've ever worked. Why? Because of the overall atmosphere of the office. My coworkers were pleasant and upbeat, as were our bosses and the people who were calling the shots. Howie himself, along with the executive producers and managers, treated everyone with respect. The staff, as far as I could tell, not only got along well but enjoyed being around one another. We even did things outside of the workplace, such as having lunches together and attending parties. Working there, I felt excited when Monday came because I wasn't bummed out that a new work week was beginning. I wasn't stressed or worried about being burned out. Who would want to be part of an organization where they often feel disrespected, unappreciated, and possibly even abused?

In contrast, much later in life, when I became a mental health professional, I worked in a therapeutic setting that was not managed properly. As a result, quite a few of my coworkers experienced tension and stress throughout the office. Many on staff were often worried about whether they would be fired and, on a few occasions, questioned whether they'd be receiving a check on payday. This created a lot of anxiety and insecurity among many who worked there, including me. These feelings were made worse by how, at times, management spoke to us using terms that were clearly threatening. At one point, they even restructured how we were paid; we were told to quit if we weren't on board with new policies. Many people ultimately did leave once they found employment elsewhere.

The two settings I just described played a significant role (for better or worse) in the staff's emotional, mental, and even physical well-being.

When it comes to difficulties with coworkers, many challenges can arise that create a toxic work environment. You've likely experienced some of these issues yourself and may be dealing with a few at this very moment. Here are some of the more common situations I've attempted to help clients with in the workplace:

- Coworkers do not get along with one another due to jealousy, gossip, a history of conflicts and arguments, or a lack of respect between them.
- Employees believe they are being treated unfairly (e.g., someone is receiving preferential treatment or is being treated more harshly than others).
- Coworkers are resentful because they feel an individual is not working hard enough, *or* they feel someone is working too much/too hard.
- A superior or coworker is bullying or harassing others, verbally or sexually.
- Employees are being discriminated against (based on sex, age, race, sexual orientation, gender, ethnicity, religion) by supervisors or people in positions of power.
- Employees feel unsafe physically, or their personal belongings are not being kept safe.

Being at a job with any of these problems can be frustrating, annoying, and stressful. But despite all these issues, a person could still find it difficult to leave—or feel forced to stay and make the best of their situation. In other words, they feel helpless or stuck.

FEELING STUCK IN A JOB

Throughout the years, I have seen clients come to therapy for the sole purpose of dealing with anxiety or stress as a result of their job. I've also experienced the challenges of providing support and examining possible solutions for someone working in a toxic environment. It would be easy for me to say to a client, "Why don't you just leave and get another job?" However, the reality is that most people can't just up and quit a job because they don't like how they're being treated or because they don't like their boss. They likely have financial obligations to their families and to themselves, which may make it difficult to simply leave. Sometimes the position that they hold may be very lucrative and they know that working somewhere else will significantly lower their income and their ability to pay their bills. Some may even be concerned about how they will be viewed by others, such as friends and family, if they quit. They may be concerned that a loved one will look down on them and question whether their decision to quit is irresponsible, thoughtless, or outright stupid.

Despite the difficulties of leaving a job, it's worth considering saying goodbye to that extremely toxic workplace or your toxic coworkers. It might be the time for you, or someone you know, to leave a place of employment, especially if it's destroying your mental and physical health. We only have one mind and one body; if we don't take care of ourselves, who will? Inner peace can be gained and a better life created if one can find the courage to make a big enough effort to find or create a better job.

When you've made the decision to leave a job, I believe it's important to do so only after you've formed a reasonable and intelligent plan and have considered all the risks. If possible, make such a move without jeopardizing your ability to manage your home, pay the bills, and support your family.

If work is the issue that brought my client in, I provide support by listening attentively and with an empathetic ear. I explore all possible plans of action and interventions that the client is open to considering. If a client feels stuck due to limited employment options (or believes they are stuck), then we must focus on managing anxiety, addressing depressive symptoms, and assisting with the mental and emotional issues that have surfaced due to their job. This usually includes exploring self-care activities they can do. I'll talk more about self-care and self-care interventions later in the book. For now, I'll say that some of the most effective self-care interventions are those that feed and nurture the mind, the body, and even the spirit.

It is my hope that by working together, I can help the client achieve the healthiest state possible, enabling them to either better deal with their situations at work or find an alternate plan, including leaving their current place of employment. Basically, I provide support for them "in the meantime" until they are able to move on to a better situation or job.

Egos and Insecurities in the Workplace

Our egos are not where we are bad but where we are wounded.

—Marianne Williamson

Whether I am listening to a client, my wife, or a friend, or reflecting on my own past job experiences, I often hear that difficulties in the workplace are the result of *egos* and *insecurities*. So often it seems that those in positions of authority demonstrate controlling, manipulative, or abusive behaviors. Sometimes the people in charge have an incredible desire to display their insights by acting as if they have all the answers or are always right. By behaving in this manner, they're demonstrating an inability to manage their *ego* and are instead feeding it.

Then there are those managers who control others as a way of hiding their weaknesses or *insecurities*. These are people who are managing in fear and are therefore afraid. Afraid of what? It varies from person to person. Perhaps they're afraid someone may discover they're not the person they're trying to present to others. Perhaps they're afraid that one day people will learn the truth: that they don't have the talent or the ability to do the job they've been assigned.

Egos and insecurities can also be seen in coworkers as well, especially in individuals who are worried about losing their jobs or being harshly judged by management, preventing them from receiving acknowledgment or recognition, thus hindering opportunities in the organization (e.g., promotions, raises).

If, however, you are a boss, manager, supervisor, commanding officer, or business owner, please consider the following. You don't have to rule with an iron fist, as if you are a dictator. Nor do you have to be rude, mean, or disrespectful in order to be an effective leader or run a successful business. You can have reasonable expectations for your staff, make them feel appreciated, and speak to them respectfully while also meeting your organization's goals.

If you are in a position of leadership, I highly recommend picking up the book *Love Works: Seven Timeless Principles for Effective Leaders* by Joel Manby. It outlines paths to success for organizations that use methods that promote respect and compassion in the workforce while creating a motivated and driven staff.[5] Even if you're not in a management position, you may still gain some insight from reading this book, especially as it relates to developing healthy relationships on the job.

THE IMPORTANCE OF BEING UNDERSTANDING IN OUR NONROMANTIC RELATIONSHIPS

Whether it's our friends, family members, or coworkers, it's extremely important to try to understand one another if we are seeking healthier relationships and more peace in our lives. So often we seem to think we understand everything about an individual or situation, perhaps because we've known someone for a long time or have been in a certain situation before. Or perhaps it's our egos telling us that we have all the answers and whatever we think is true.

Sometimes we feel we know a person or a situation because of either our own beliefs or those we've inherited from our parents or the media. However, many times we are simply ignorant when it comes to truly understanding another human being, regardless of the role they play in our lives. How can we know the inner struggles that another person deals with on a regular basis? How can we know how much love a person is truly capable of displaying? Or how much hurt and pain they may be dealing with? Most of us are struggling to even understand ourselves.

Our own ignorance of others has often made us quick to judge someone, which can negatively impact our ability to foster healthy relationships. Being critical of something or someone based solely on our limited perspective would be like saying an apple tree is diseased because it produced one or two rotten apples when there may be a variety of reason why this has occurred. It's important to look at the entire tree—that is, to look at a person in their entirety. It can be very harmful and even destructive to our relationships if we define a person based on one statement they made or one action they did, ignoring the totality of their life and being.

It would be more beneficial if we put effort into trying

to understand other people, other communities, other races, other nations, other religions, and the struggles others may have experienced. No one has all the answers. I've always felt that true wisdom is knowing and accepting that neither you nor I know everything. I wish we could accept that there will always be different perspectives. We, as egotistical humans, will never agree with everything someone says or does (and often for good reasons). The people we interact with on a regular basis will eventually do something that doesn't make sense to us. If we can't try to understand or at least relate to the experiences of others, their points of view, and especially their pain, it will definitely make growing together difficult—as a family, community, nation, or planet.

I have a saying that I often use: "Ego divides; spirit unites." We are either living within our individual egos or living in spirit. It's extremely difficult to live in both at the same time. When we are *living in our ego*, our primary focus is satisfying ourselves, getting what we want, putting ourselves first, and being right. However, when we *live in spirit*, we are focused on taking care of and being there for others. Living in spirit allows us to feel more connected, more united, and more at peace with others (and likely ourselves as well). Living in ego is what drives billion-dollar corporations to make excessive amounts of money without caring for those who have less. On the other hand, an example of living in spirit is when people come together using their time, energy, and resources to feed the hungry. Living in ego is why we have wars, dictators, and different religions judging or despising one another. Living in spirit allows families and communities to accept and love one another unconditionally, regardless of differences.

Trying to better understand our family members, friends, classmates, coworkers, and even our rivals will likely go a long way toward having more meaningful interactions and relationships. These improved connections with one another will go a long way toward reducing the loneliness that so many experience today.

CHAPTER 5

Lessons Learned About Men and Therapy

It's easier to build strong children than to repair broken men.

—Frederick Douglass

As a kid growing up on the South Side of Chicago, I don't ever recall hearing the word *therapy* or the phrase *mental health treatment*. I was familiar with the term *psychiatrist*, but my understanding was that's who people go to see when they're "crazy." Any other problems you might face, you simply push through them. If you absolutely, positively need to go talk to someone (and your friends or family can't be the listening ear), you should find the courage to go speak with your minister or pastor.

The ages nine through nineteen were an extremely

emotionally challenging period for me. There were many times when I felt totally inadequate, unattractive, and like I didn't fit in with my peers. I felt like such an outsider that I remember writing a poem in class one day called "This World Is Not My Home." It was about how I believed I must be from another planet because it seemed so hard trying to belong, be happy, and exist here.

I also recall being thirteen years old and having a pretty serious crush on a girl who clearly didn't feel the same about me. I was so distraught that I started questioning if I even wanted to live anymore! Looking back, I can identify this as dramatic thinking—all because a girl didn't like me! But I was clearly young, hurting, and dealing with the emotional insecurities of an adolescent.

This was a period in my life when having someone I could talk to would have been so beneficial to me, especially if it would've been a supportive, positive older male. I'm not saying an older female could not have played this role for me, but I grew up exclusively with my mother and older sister, and I was definitely not comfortable talking to them about my issues. Therefore, as a growing adolescent, I didn't have many options when I wanted to seek out someone for advice.

When it came to getting advice, I would most often turn to my male friends. They knew about as much as I did, which was next to nothing when it came to life, relationships, feelings, or personal challenges.

I didn't have a relationship with my father, nor did I have a father figure like a big brother, a mentor, a grandfather, or even an uncle to confide in. (I technically had an uncle, but he wasn't the greatest communicator. Plus, we rarely saw each other.) As a result, I did what so many other young men do when they're struggling with their thoughts, their emotions, and their lives. I dealt with my pain on my own. This would have been a great time to learn about therapists (or at least to find wise and experienced people to talk to) and the benefits that can come from having someone to process my thoughts and feelings with. This also would have been a great time to be introduced to the idea of therapy and the value it could provide for me then and in the future as well.

WHY THE FOCUS ON MEN?

There are several reasons why I wanted to write a chapter that focuses exclusively on men. First, I am far more aware of the emotional, mental, and societal challenges that a male may be forced to deal with in today's world. Second, women have a greater ability to know when they're struggling and then seek assistance—in the form of friends, therapists, family members, and so on.

Another reason, and what's really unfortunate, is how frequently men are the impetus behind many of my female clients (regardless of age) going into therapy in the first place. So often women are hurt by the words and actions of men. More than 90 percent of my female clients (both adults and adolescents) are in treatment because of negative experiences they've had with men. Some common themes include being physically, sexually, or emotionally abused by a man; being emotionally or physically distant from a father or father figure; being mistreated or disrespected by a male in the workplace; being pressured, teased, or victimized by males in school or work; and reexamining toxic relationships.

A chapter on men is also necessary due to the percentage of men who are in positions of leadership or power and who make a significant impact (positive or negative) on those around them. In most settings, the role that an influential male plays in the world is too great to be ignored. Too often, those in positions of power (which also applies to females) become addicted to it and obsessed with obtaining more. In doing so, the fair and ethical treatment of others is sacrificed. "With great power comes great responsibility" is an adage that's been quoted by many and has even been thrust into pop culture when Peter Parker's Uncle Ben uttered it in *Spider-Man*.[1] But I can't help but wonder what percentage of men in positions of power (both in their communities and homes) are truly striving to be responsible, moral, and ethical toward those around them and those they will likely impact. Men warrant a whole chapter (if not complete books) in order to better understand them, their tendencies, their unresolved issues, their pain, the societal challenges they have to navigate, and the need many of them have to understand themselves.

GETTING MEN TO SEE A THERAPIST

This will likely come as no surprise, but men seek mental health services far less than women. According to the National Center for Health Statistics' *National Health Interview Survey 2020*, 25.6 percent of women receive mental health treatment during a twelve-month period compared to 14.6 percent of men.[2] Now let's consider how many people, especially men, who would likely benefit from getting mental health treatment yet don't consider doing so.

When a heterosexual couple has their first appointment with me, one of the questions I ultimately end up asking is, "Whose idea was it to come to therapy?" The vast majority of the time it was not the man's choice. However, if the man was the initiator, there are several possible reasons why. First, he may actually have a desire to heal or fix the relationship. This is great and what I hope is the case. Then there are times when the man thinks it will satisfy her, or maybe it'll be enough to get her off his back because she's been suggesting therapy for the longest time. On a few occasions, the man's partner has made some sort of ultimatum that they go speak to a counselor.

THE IMPORTANCE OF MEN WORKING ON THEMSELVES

We should all work on our minds, bodies, and spirits on a regular basis. This is true if we want to be the best possible versions of ourselves, and even more so for men, considering the impact (positive or negative) that they can have on people and society.

When men fail to invest the time and energy into working on themselves, they run the risk of leaving issues unresolved, and of their emotional wounds hurting those around them. Men who have unhealed wounds tend to be angry; lack patience, understanding, and empathy; and often find it difficult to engage in nurturing, healthy relationships (with friends, family, or significant others). When men fail to work on themselves, they hamper their ability to heal and grow. I'm concerned for all the broken men in the world who display maladaptive behaviors and make bad choices where those around them will ultimately pay the price for their unresolved issues.

WHY ARE MEN RESISTANT TO THERAPY?

Every man has his reasons for not wanting to seek mental health therapy. Every man is entitled to have his opinions about treatment, and some may be valid. However, male or female, we all experience challenges and sometimes need help for ourselves or with our relationships.

One reason men tend *not* to seek counseling is the pressure that society places on them and what it means to be a man. I'm confident that a lot of men believe that going to see a clinician is an indication that something is inherently wrong with them. That somehow they are flawed, broken, and too weak to handle the adversity life has thrown their way. Our world, through many different avenues (our beliefs, our expectations, the media), seems to have communicated to them that strength should be displayed at all times, and anything less than that means a man is weak. I'll discuss the pressure society places on men more in a moment.

Another reason men may be reluctant to consider therapy is their egos. People, especially men, have a strong desire to be right. Right about what's best for themselves, right about what's best for others, right about what's best for society, and right about what's best for the world. A man may believe that going to see a licensed clinician makes him appear as though he doesn't know the best course of action or how to resolve a conflict. I believe being strong enough to admit there are things you don't know (or areas you should work on) is a sign of wisdom and demonstrates a willingness to be honest with yourself.

Some men are not only resistant to therapy but also reluctant to look inside and do the work that may lead to personal growth, insight, and healing.

Ask yourself this: Who is likely to go to a self-improvement retreat, read a self-help book, go to a seminar to better themselves, attend church services, join a book club, or be part of a meditation or yoga group? Of course, there are plenty of men who would and do engage in these activities. However, I believe in most cases you would agree that women tend to do these things much more often than men. The point is that women are more inclined than men to seek out whatever interventions are necessary in order to better their lives, continue their personal evolution, and heal their inner wounds.

Societal Pressures Defining What a Man Should Be

Today's culture is constantly emphasizing what "a real man" (or a *high-value* man) is or isn't. This includes what he should look like, how he should conduct his business, and the type of lifestyle he should have. Society often expects "real" men to be physically strong, mentally tough, and powerful, which often refers to their social status and financial worth. Society also defines a "manly man" as someone who is fit, attractive, tall, well groomed, and a sharp dresser. Being muscular or in shape is definitely considered a plus. Modern culture dictates that a man should carry himself in a way that hovers somewhere between confident and flirty, bordering on outright arrogant. Real men are also supposed to be extremely proficient, well endowed, and satisfying in the bedroom. For some, real men are wealthy, hold positions of authority, and have a certain amount of notoriety or fame. There are plenty of men who strive to meet these goals, and inherently there's nothing wrong with this, but they shouldn't be requirements to be considered a real man.

When you think about some of the characteristics I just described, it's no wonder we often idolize rock stars, actors, and athletes. For many, someone like Dwayne "The Rock" Johnson would easily check a lot of the boxes for what's considered a real man in today's world.

However, for the vast majority of men, the traits described above are often unrealistic. As a result, these ideals can add a lot of pressure to his life as he tries to reach them and receive the respect he wants. Not meeting these aspirations can cause some men to feel *less-than* as they unfortunately compare themselves to those who appear to *have it all*.

It is quite common for men to feel unable to express what may be considered weakness. This means appearing emotionally, mentally, and maybe even physically strong pretty much at all times. I've actually heard men say when they look at other men who are crying (even if they're celebrating a great accomplishment) that they're "looking weak." Apparently, the false message is that no matter what the situation, men shouldn't appear emotional, uncertain, or fearful. Men often feel that if they express vulnerability or weakness in any form, they'll likely be judged, criticized, or condemned. If they display these traits openly and frequently, they may question themselves or their acceptance in society, whether women are going to find them desirable, whether employers are going to want to hire them, and whether they are going to be respected by other men. These questions are what cause a man to go through life wearing a mask, trying to be someone he isn't.

Some men go through life feeling invisible because they don't believe they measure up to what women want or what society expects. For a large portion of my life, it seemed to me that women would often say they wanted a "nice guy" only to find themselves in relationships with guys who were anything but. The nice guys typically don't represent some of the characteristics I previously mentioned, nor do they always have the necessary confidence or experience when it comes to approaching women. As a result, many men are easily overlooked, undervalued, underappreciated, or not even given a chance by women. I know this is how I felt during high school and for a portion of my young adulthood, when I was labeled the "nice guy" while repeatedly seeing women around me be drawn to toxic men, also known as the "bad boys." This feeling of inadequacy, of not measuring up, can easily make men susceptible to becoming frustrated, lonely, and depressed.

These expectations for men can sometimes lead to what's called "toxic masculinity." This is where the pressure to meet the stereotypical traits of how a man should be causes him to act in ways that are potentially negative or harmful to himself, those around him, the community, and the world.

Examples of toxic masculinity can be seen when males of any age bully or try to control others. They may feel justified in frequently expressing anger and aggression, looking for opportunities to show their superiority through fighting or brandishing their guns. Some may display selfishness or an "all about me" attitude. They may avoid demonstrating empathy or compassion for others (or they are unable to), especially toward women. Some men with a high level of toxic masculinity may place an overemphasis on acquiring material things (regardless of what it takes to get them). There are also those men who demonstrate this mindset by using women for money, material things, a place to live, or simply as sexual objects. Within this mindset, women are seen as something to possess, making a man feel superior and feeding his ego.

Before going any further, I would like to point out that just because *masculinity* is placed after the word *toxic*, it does not mean that the stereotypical behaviors described above are reserved strictly for men. There appears to be a case for "toxic femininity" as well. This can be observed in women who misuse, control, or take advantage of men. The bottom line here is that anyone, male or female, can be toxic, especially if they feel the need to measure up to society's expectations or be in a position of power.

From a very early age, the message conveyed to young boys (me included) is very different from the one that is conveyed to young girls. When a boy is growing up, it probably won't be long before he starts hearing phrases like "Big boys don't cry" when he falls down and scrapes his knee. As he gets a little older, he may start hearing statements such as "Suck it up!" "Man up!" "Don't be soft!" or "Don't be a p---y!" I believe by the time the typical male has reached eighteen years of age, he has received countless messages from a variety of sources that have told him to keep his emotions in check (i.e., buried inside)—perhaps with the exception of anger or toughness.

Showing other less aggressive emotions may make him look weak.

Meanwhile, little girls are often encouraged to communicate their feelings: "Share your emotions." "Express what's going on inside." "Be open and transparent." "Be vulnerable." Although the expectation to be strong may be increasing for women in society, if they do happen to show their feelings or become emotional, people may chalk it up to them being female.

Being encouraged from an early age to bottle up their emotions (in order to avoid appearing weak) has produced a lot of males who are now conditioned to avoid addressing the true source of their pain. The individuals I see in my personal life, in society, and in my office minimize their issues in an effort to appear as if they have everything under control. When asked if they're okay or struggling, they respond by saying, "I got this!" "I'm fine," "I'm okay," or "I'm good." Repressing something that needs to be addressed does not make a person strong, nor does it make the problem go away.

As a therapist working with men and being male myself, I think it's important to acknowledge the ideals that society and the media impose upon us to define modern manhood. How often do we pick up messages in movies, TV shows, or music that a man should demonstrate his toughness by talking tough, enacting revenge, fighting, or pulling out a weapon? I don't see how anyone could be surprised by the amount of violence that takes place at the hands of men in our world, especially in the United States (particularly in major cities).

Every day, men, especially men of color, are shot and killed in this country—often senselessly. As a result, not only are lives lost, but families and communities are devastated as they mourn another unnecessary death. Whether it be an altercation in the streets, domestic violence within the home, or a mass shooter in a public setting, how often is the perpetrator a man? Violence taking place at the hands of men will continue at unfortunate rates until society decides to actively address the matter and men consciously work on themselves, heal, and make wise choices that improve our world.

Women Contributing to a Man's Insecurities

There are times in which the woman is contributing to the man's insecurities, weaknesses, and fears. She may be doing this knowingly, or she may be clueless as to how her actions or words are negatively impacting him.

A man in a relationship may have some valid underlying reasons for his self-doubt or lack of confidence, including family-of-origin issues or his romantic past. One example is a couple who is living together or married; perhaps she's the primary breadwinner or the only one employed at the moment. Of course, this isn't her fault, but some men in this position may question their manhood for not being able to provide for her or the family.

Maybe she frequently criticizes him about what he does, what he says, how little money he makes, and what he hasn't accomplished. If she is (or if he believes she is) frequently talking down to him, as if he's a child, or if she is being disrespectful, he may become defensive and annoyed, if not outright angry. If the woman has a very strong personality and is very accomplished, he may even feel emasculated.

For men who have anger issues or lack of self-restraint, it's an unfortunate possibility that they can become verbally abusive or even physically aggressive. Hopefully, things never escalate to the point where someone's safety or physical health is at risk. Let me make this extremely clear: I believe no matter how mistreated a man may feel in a relationship, he is never justified in being violent. If a man gets to a point where he wants to put his hands on his partner because of what she says or does, it is time to consider either going to therapy or walking away from the relationship altogether. Of course, there are instances in which the female is the abuser. Abuse in this situation is also inappropriate.

Women may also contribute to the frustrations and insecurities of a man *unknowingly*. Perhaps she's passionate about her beliefs and thinks that what she's doing is in the best interest of their relationship or family. Some women who've experienced painful or toxic outcomes in previous relationships spend a lot of energy trying to prevent similar issues from happening again.

Then there are women who have become accustomed to taking care of themselves; after spending years on their own, they may struggle with sharing the decision-making process. In these situations, I strongly encourage my female clients to realize that if they are in a serious, committed relationship, they are part of a team. Teams have a much greater chance of success if members are able to work together, when each person is able to play their specific position. Strong team members tend to accept and understand the strengths and weaknesses of those on their side. Finally, it can be extremely important to create a space for the man to be a man. Leave room for him to play his part; this may mean respecting his input and in certain situations letting him make the final decision.

Positive Male Representation—or the Lack Thereof

Now let's talk about male images that are typically *not* emphasized or rarely even discussed. Take a moment and compare how often men are portrayed as aggressive and violent to how often they are portrayed as kind, generous, sensitive, and thoughtful. I rarely hear about a man recognized, discussed, or praised for displaying these traits. If he did, it's likely he'd be considered "soft," a "beta male," or labeled as gay. How often do you hear young boys or men talking about how they want to be more like Gandhi, Bishop Desmond Tutu, Albert Einstein, Nelson Mandela, former congressman John Lewis, or Martin Luther King Jr.? These men are admired and looked up to, but it seems very few men aspire to be like them today. In today's world, these men do not represent the ideals of strength, toughness, or success, but they probably should. However, in the twenty-first century, perhaps if these men were also MMA fighters; had great wealth; talked tough; excelled in a sport; or were rappers, A-list actors, YouTube influencers, or politicians, other males would try to emulate them.

Despite men as a group being more reluctant to go to therapy, there does appear to be some progress in this area. More and more male celebrities and professional athletes have willingly come forward and shared their personal struggles with mental health issues. The more these men, whom society idolizes, share their decisions to seek treatment, the more the idea of seeing a therapist will become normalized. This will hopefully result in more men taking the chance and going to get the help they need.

MALE MINORITIES IN TREATMENT

> *It will be found that men see evil in those who differ from them, good in those who agree with them. The man who greatly loves himself and is enamored of his opinions will love all those who agree with him and dislike those who disagree with him.*
>
> —James Allen

I believe that whatever our society is struggling with, it's going to be exponentially worse, or at the very least more challenging, for a man of color. Therefore it's warranted to discuss the issues that male minorities have to deal with in today's world and how beneficial it could be for us all to better understand their journey. As a therapist, I also believe that it's imperative that my fellow mental health professionals try their best to realize the additional societal issues that minority men may encounter by considering their experiences from a historical perspective and how the past may be affecting them now.

Many non-White men and minorities, at some point in their lives, have likely had to deal with experiences that include not being given fair or equal opportunities, not feeling seen, not feeling heard, being viewed as inferior, being paid less for a job or task, being feared based on their skin color, being prejudged, being misunderstood, or simply being avoided altogether.

In many economically challenged communities (typically found in large cities), minorities, both male or female, are forced to deal with substandard living conditions, challenges associated with not speaking the language of the majority, high crime rates, a lack of resources, the presence of drug and alcohol abuse, low-paying jobs, and education systems that are not on par with suburban or private schools.

Struggles of the American Indian and the African American

Two communities I am personally worried about in the United States are American Indians and African American or Black males. Of course, I'm also concerned about the challenges that African American females and other minorities have to deal with. However, I believe that in this country, these two groups appear to have struggled the most when trying to assimilate and be an accepted part of this nation while simultaneously trying to recover from the atrocities that were part of their past. In many ways, the American Indians and African American men still show the residual effects of a history of oppression.

Even today, in the twenty-first century, some people are still unfairly judged by their race, religion, nationality, socioeconomic status, gender, or sexual orientation. This is especially true with African American men and American Indians. Many writers have delved deep into their challenges and experiences. However, for this portion of the book, I will simply share my thoughts and experiences working with and being around men of color.

For the sake of transparency, I've not had the opportunity to work with an American Indian. However, throughout my life, starting in college, I've spent time learning about their stories and their trials.

Many American Indians have struggled for generations with a variety of challenges, often while being confined to life on a reservation. This group of people had their land taken away and were relocated, and countless were killed—all while facing various abuses throughout their history. As a result, this group of proud people continues to struggle in a variety of ways: inadequate health care, voting challenges, high unemployment rates, substandard housing, violence (often against women and children), limited educational opportunities, poverty, and high rates of addiction and suicide. It is my hope that one day their circumstances will improve dramatically, that this underserved community will finally get their needs met, and that I will be able to help in some way as well.

African American Men: Their History,
Identity, and Desire for Respect

There's an old saying in the African American community: "When White folks catch a cold, Black people catch the flu."

No matter what problems society at large may be dealing with—whether it's economics, food shortages, educational shortcomings, health disparity, or crime and violence—it's likely to be far worse for Black people.

When discussing Black men in therapy, I believe it's beneficial, if not necessary, to start with the past. Many people are aware of the dark time in US history when Africans were forcibly taken from their homeland and brought to America during the transatlantic slave trade. I have seen data suggesting over twelve million Africans were brought against their will to the US during that time. In addition to being taken from their native country, they were deprived of their culture, their language, their families, and their identities.

The amount of trauma—physical, emotional, and spiritual—that both the African man and woman experienced being brought to this country is incalculable. Imagine the suffering they endured when they were taken away from the only land that they knew to come here to be treated like animals, potentially being tortured or killed. Having to deal with these atrocities went on to deeply affect African Americans for generations.

In many ways, the impact of enslavement can still be felt today in the form of discrimination and prejudice. I will acknowledge that significant advancements have been made throughout the decades. And yet, despite this progress, in the twenty-first century there are still those who consider people of color or minorities to be inferior to their majority counterparts.

Despite being forcibly taken from her home, the African woman was, in some ways, able to hold on to at least one part of her identity (although not always): being able to be a mother. Being able to give birth, feed, and nurture a new life.

Regrettably, the African man was unable to hold on to a label in which he could feel a sense of pride. He may have been allowed to impregnate another slave, but it's very unlikely he would have been able to be a father—at least not in the way he would've wanted to be. As time went on, even after slavery ended, the Black man had to fight for everything: food, homes, property, the right to vote, the right to be educated, jobs, human rights, respect, and decency.

Despite slavery taking place so long ago, it often appears to me that many African American men still feel as if they are fighting to be treated fairly, have equal opportunities, and be respected. Many are trying to figure out their identity—who they are within their own families, communities, this country, and the world. Many African American men feel like society is against them, always trying to prevent them from making it in this world. Some feel that, in order to accomplish their goals, they are forced to work harder, focus more, be more self-disciplined, and be smarter than those of other races. And then there are those who feel that they are entitled to have the life they want and will therefore use whatever means they deem necessary to get it (regardless of how harmful it may be to others).

When people, regardless of their race, are not sure who they are or how they fit into this world, frustration, confusion, depression, and pain are likely to set in.

Personally and professionally, I've seen many men, especially African American men, who have a strong desire to be valued, appreciated, and respected. Some try to gain these things by working hard and hopefully creating a successful career, whereas other men try to gain notoriety or attention in the hopes that their achievements will allow them to be seen and noticed.

Some men have a tendency to pursue things in order to gain attention. There have been instances in which men have sought wealth by acquiring a job or position that puts them in the limelight (athlete, actor, singer/rap artist, politician, etc.), while others have focused on their exterior by building a great physique or being impeccably groomed. There have been men who do things such as choosing a vehicle that they believe represents a certain status, joining a fraternity, becoming part of a gang, or many other things in order to be noticed. I am in no way saying that *all* men pursue these things just to gain attention. Some men who pursue these things are sincere about their interests and their passions. For them, obtaining success, taking care of their families, or leaving a legacy is the ultimate goal, and the attention gained along the way is simply an additional plus. For others, it may finally provide some of the validation they've spent so much of their lives seeking.

Working with African American Men in Therapy

As a therapist, I believe listening to understand, without judgment, is necessary to serve any client but perhaps even more so if the client is a minority. If the client is an African American man, gaining a grasp of their perspective and personal history is crucial to helping them with whatever challenge they've brought to the session. When a mental health professional has an African American male client, the mental health professional should ask appropriate, pertinent questions to gain an understanding of their client's struggles, their experiences, their desires, and their pain, along with what brought them to therapy in the first place. Gaining understanding is vital to providing care and support, especially if the therapist is not a minority. Doing this will likely go a long way in developing a healthy, positive, trusting therapeutic relationship.

Some African American men have a lot of distrust toward the health care system. I, too, have questioned the medical community, with an additional degree of cynicism as a Black man. I once was in a situation where a White male doctor was causing me significant pain, and it didn't appear that he cared—he never apologized, nor did he try to ease up—which made me question whether he was intentionally hurting me because of the color of my skin.

This lack of trust is the result of a long history in America of African Americans being discriminated against, exploited, and mistreated by those who work in medicine. Therefore it is necessary that a White therapist gain the trust of an African American client, even if it takes time to develop. I believe the depth of a relationship can be seen in the amount of trust that exists between people. So if the therapist is successful in establishing a solid rapport with him, doors may be opened, allowing the client and clinician to address a variety of issues. Topics that may help the African American client with accomplishing goals include looking inside himself, better understanding who he is, better understanding what he wants for his life, becoming more aware of his emotional/mental wounds, learning ways to address his past pains or trauma, and creating new thought patterns. Hopefully, the therapist can help him resolve the issues that brought him to therapy and develop positive behaviors, make better life choices, and see what's possible for himself and his relationships.

THE ABSENCE OF AN EMOTIONALLY HEALTHY MALE ROLE MODEL

It's unfortunate when anyone—African American or otherwise, male or female—grows up without the influence of a well-adjusted, mentally healthy, balanced man in their life. I, like many others, was raised without my father. This could very well have been a blessing due to my earliest memories of him being emotionally detached, controlling, easily angered, and abusive, with a tendency to overindulge in alcohol—topped off with a good helping of narcissism. When I was about eight years old, my mother, sister, and I were eventually able to escape a very toxic environment. (We literally packed up what we needed and, without telling anyone, moved to another area of Chicago while he was at work.) Unfortunately, a lot of mental and emotional damage took place that mostly impacted my mother and sister because they were the primary targets of his abuse. Looking back on my early childhood, I believe that my late father was simply incapable of knowing how to nurture any relationship, had unresolved anger issues, was selfish, and was functional alcoholic.

My mother remarried in my early teens; however, she chose yet another man with a *very*—and I do mean *very*—questionable character. I won't get into too much detail, but I will say that despite seeing him every day, he never became a father figure to me. There was never any true connection. I'm pretty sure he didn't care about me, and the feeling was mutual due to the way I felt he treated my mother. I'm not proud to share this, nor do I condone violence; however, as a young adult there were a couple of occasions where we came pretty close to getting into a physical altercation.

When I reflect on the past, I firmly believe that neither he nor my biological father was an emotionally healthy man. I didn't gain anything from the men I grew up with, but I was able to see the type of man I was determined *not* to become. How many other young men grew up the way I did, without a father, a father figure, or an older man to pull us under his wings and provide guidance, support, and affection?

I think it's extremely important that young men have older men in their lives who can demonstrate what it means to be a man with morals, values, principles, courage, and a good heart. Without older men serving in these roles, what happens to the next generation of boys? I believe this produces young men who will crave that fatherly connection they never had. When they're older they may struggle with being a present parent themselves because they have no idea what an emotionally healthy father looks like, increasing the chances that they will take their pain and resentment out on others. And finally, without a father, father figure, or mentor to guide them, men may make choices that produce negative consequences, including passing on dysfunctional family behaviors to future generations.

Finding Role Models in the Community

I was a senior in high school when I became aware of the void that existed in the lives of many young men. There I was, crammed into a car with five other guys. I'm not sure if I made the statement or someone else did, but as we rode down the street, we realized that none of us grew up with or had a relationship with our fathers. Once we all acknowledged this unfortunate truth, we all pledged that if we were to one day have children of our own, even if we did not get along or remain with the mother, we would do everything in our power to be a father to those kids. We would give to them what we were unable to experience ourselves.

It's important to understand the challenges young men face when they grow up without a healthy and positive father (or father figure) in their lives. I purposefully stated "healthy" and "positive" due to the unfortunate fact that just because a father is physically present does not mean he is emotionally present. I've had multiple young clients (boys and girls) who, despite being raised with their dads, feel no sense of connection to him. Some were even abused by their dads. Often these fathers don't spend time with them, don't understand how to communicate with them, or are unable to nurture a quality relationship. In these situations, I can't help but wonder, *Are they just being the father that they saw when they were growing up?*

When no healthy father or father figure is present for a boy or young man, a great opportunity is created for someone—a willing, stable, emotionally healthy male—to step in and serve as a mentor, role model, life coach, or surrogate father. This person can prove to be very beneficial to a young person's overall development. Hopefully, through this relationship the young person can gain insight from the man by learning new ways to overcome challenges, developing resiliency, and creating and achieving goals. Ideally, the boy, adolescent, or young man would see the importance of respecting others as well as himself. They would also learn how to treat the women in their lives, both now and in the future. If they've never experienced it before, they'll now have the opportunity to see that a man can be supportive, nurturing, and loving—yet still strong. This relationship can become a "corrective experience," where they can see what's possible, despite the history of negativity, toxicity, or absenteeism they may have experienced with men from their past. Just having someone there to spend quality time with or engage in conversation can be extremely impactful and lead to amazing changes in a young person's daily life and in their future.

There are a variety of ways in which young boys or teenagers can receive mentorship. Some may be lucky enough to have such a person in their family (an uncle, a grandparent, or an older cousin). Sometimes mentors can be found within the school through a caring teacher, counselor, or coach. Programs such as Big Brothers Big Sisters of America can be found simply by doing a Google search. Despite the availability of these programs, I believe we need more. Perhaps we can develop mentorship programs within our schools. Churches (especially megachurches), businesses, and other public organizations could also step up and do a lot more to help our young men reach their full potential. Everything we do to try to help our youth (especially males) will produce amazing benefits for our communities.

I believe having a father figure or mentor is so important that even in my fifties, I still would love to have such a person in my life—someone whom I could turn to for advice, vent to, engage in good conversation with, or gain some additional perspective from. Someone with whom I can talk about a variety of topics, from sports, to politics, to life, to marriage, or someone I can simply sit down and play a game of chess with. I am still looking for this relationship, and one day I hope to find it. It's sad for me to admit this, but I've never felt important in the eyes of an older man, nor do I recall ever hearing an older adult male (even my father) tell me that he loves me. As unfortunate as that may sound, I know there are many others who also share this experience. It is my hope and prayer that men continue to grow and evolve, becoming more in touch with who they are on the inside, and that they are able to heal their wounds, ultimately becoming a source of love for so many who truly desire that from them.

Other Positive Influences

Positive role models and mentors don't always have to be men, and they don't always need to be physically present. Whether we like to admit it or not, many young men look up to the people they frequently see, which include athletes, actors, singers, and rap artists. I'm sure there are those who have a problem with these individuals being so admired, and I totally get it. But I don't believe there's anything wrong with a young man finding someone they admire and emulating that person's life or accomplishments. It's okay as long as the person they're looking up to encourages people to be better versions of themselves and to make a positive difference in the lives of others, not engage in toxic or illegal behaviors, and not cause others harm. Knowing that it's very common for popular individuals to become substitute role models, I hope young men will also be exposed and open to identifying men who are *not* part of the entertainment/sports industry.

Since my father wasn't around to raise me, the late Walter Payton, former running back for the Chicago Bears, was my first role model (not counting Spider-Man). I often read about how hard he worked at practice and how well liked he was by his teammates; ultimately, I saw how he was able to accomplish amazing things in his life. Unfortunately, once I got to my late teens and early twenties, I don't recall looking up to any man or having anyone serve as an example for me. However, during my late twenties and early thirties, I became exposed to several authors and motivational speakers whose words had a significant impact on me and helped me understand more effective ways of thinking, accomplishing goals, and growing spiritually.

I clearly remember being so impressed by the energy and inspirational words of Tony Robbins (coach, speaker, and author) during late-night infomercials that I purchased his entire audiocassette series. I went on to be exposed to other men with positive messages, including the late Wayne Dyer, Dennis Kimbro, and Les Brown. At different points in my life, these men became my mentors. Even now I still strive to discover individuals who inspire me to grow and gain insight from their speeches, videos, seminars, and books.

Male Friendships—or the Lack Thereof

In addition to role models, a man's relationships with other men can be extremely valuable when it comes to their mental and emotional health. By having quality relationships with other men (or at least *one* other man), men gain someone they can turn to for ideas, advice, or a good time; someone they can share personal challenges with; and someone whom they can relate to who is also a male.

Unfortunately, *not* having these connections can be detrimental. A lot of men find it difficult to develop relationships with other males. It's very common that the close relationships guys have with one another were formed in grade school, high school, or college. However, it is possible to make these connections in adulthood through work, extracurricular activities, or mutual friends. Unfortunately, the odds of this happening significantly decrease as men get older.

As men age, they may be reluctant or find it difficult to develop new connections with other males. Reasons this can become challenging include men requiring a significant amount of time for trust to be developed, not having similar interests or lifestyles, and, as briefly discussed in chapter 4, not wanting another guy to think they are gay.

Personally, despite wanting a closer connection to guys, I have found it difficult to nurture healthy relationships and spend quality time with other men. I believe this is due to a variety of reasons, including leaving my hometown and moving to a different part of the country, not once but twice. As a result, my male friends and I gradually saw and spoke to one another less often. I still remain close to them, and from time to time I will connect on the phone and enjoy a good laugh or share some stimulating conversation.

If you're reading this and you are a male who would like to build friendships with other men, I encourage you to consider joining various social groups and engaging in activities that may provide an opportunity to develop new relationships (martial arts, sports leagues, theater groups, chess clubs, etc.). These activities can benefit men by reducing or eliminating the isolation and loneliness they, including myself, often have had to deal with.

MEN HEALING THEMSELVES

A man should intentionally strive to heal and grow. His impact on society and those around him is undeniable. Men play a significant role in whether our communities and homes are safe and loving or filled with fear and volatility. I hope that men are honest enough with themselves to admit that, regardless of where they are in their lives, there is always more internal work they can do in order to remain or become better versions of themselves. This work typically involves making a sincere effort to invest in nurturing one's mind, body, and spirit—areas that are discussed deeply in the upcoming chapter on self-care.

Interventions and Tools for Men

As a mental health professional, when I start my workday, I am often excited when I see that a man is among my scheduled clients. Women, couples, and children make up a significant portion of those I provide therapy for. I am grateful when anyone has trusted me to be their therapist to help them deal with their personal challenges. However, when that client is a man, first, I am proud of the fact that he was able to acknowledge he needed help while also being strong enough to make and keep his appointment. Second, I feel blessed with the opportunity to help a fellow man and impact his life, possibly assisting him with getting stronger in areas such as self-discipline, self-control, resiliency, finding peace, finding acceptance, letting go/surrendering, and being more loving, forgiving, and kind. If we are successful in improving these areas, a ripple effect will occur, allowing his progress to spread out and touch others who are a part of his world.

There is no one way to promote inner growth and healing,

but I do believe it's beneficial to consider all possibilities. There are many tools and interventions that I encourage men to consider. Growth and healing can come from reading insightful, inspirational, or motivational books; watching videos; journaling; and attending self-help seminars, retreats, and even uplifting religious services. Men can also work on themselves by taking the time to reflect when alone, perhaps by exploring the benefits of meditation or yoga. Taking care of their bodies by eating healthy foods and getting sufficient sleep cannot be underestimated when it comes to supporting their mental and emotional health. He may also benefit from doing simple things, like laughing as much as possible, having healthy and positive relationships, and going to see a mental health clinician if need be.

I begin every day by reading something that will feed my mind and spirit for one hour. I then transition to doing twenty to thirty minutes of meditation, followed by another twenty minutes of yoga. Anything that opens a doorway to healing and growth, no matter how large or small, will likely yield positive results for both men and the people they impact.

CHAPTER 6

Lessons Learned About Children and Adolescents

When a flower doesn't bloom you fix the environment in which it grows, not the flower.

—Alexander den Heijer

While living in Southern California, I worked at a day-treatment facility where children with severe emotional and mental health issues attended a weekly five-day program after school. This program had vans and drivers that would travel throughout South Central Los Angeles and bring them to a place where they would first have a snack, and then break out into their age-appropriate groups. Later, they would receive individual and/or group therapy. These children, ranging from five to twelve years old, could be very challenging. Some of them would become so out of control that they needed to be restrained or placed in designated time-out rooms to keep them from hurting themselves or someone else, or to just give them a quiet place to calm down.

One day a caring foster mother brought me a six-year-old girl who had a host of behavioral, emotional, and mental health issues. She was in major need of speech therapy (which often made it extremely difficult to know what she was trying to say when she did decide to speak). She was capable of extreme and sudden mood changes during which she could become physically aggressive to the point where bystanders might end up being scratched or bitten. In addition to all this, she was also a victim of significant sexual abuse. I will not disclose the greater depth of her issues and behaviors, but know that they clearly demonstrated that at least one adult had taken advantage of her, leaving her deeply scarred.

Despite her history and volatile behaviors, this innocent, damaged six-year-old and I developed a connection, so much so that while in day treatment she often preferred to be with me all afternoon (something that was not always possible, as I had other child clients as well). Despite the significant challenges that she presented to the staff and myself, and regardless of her improvements, one day the well-intentioned foster parent informed me that this little girl's time was about to run out: if we couldn't do more for her quicker, she would be returned to the foster system and in need of a new placement. Unfortunately, that is what ultimately happened. I'll never forget the last evening I saw her. I did the best I could to explain to her how important it was that she continue to try to control her outbursts, make better choices, and not hurt others. Then I said my final goodbye to this young spirit, whom I felt both responsible for and attached to (as I tried to hold back the tears that were forming in my eyes). I was so disappointed in myself because I felt like I didn't do what I needed to do. I was unable to save her. I didn't help her quickly enough. I didn't heal her. In the end, I felt as if I was the reason for her returning to the foster system.

I mention this story as an extreme example of how much damage adults can do to children. Yes, this is a unique case, but whether we are a parent, teacher, relative, family friend, counselor, or neighbor, the things we do and say to children have lasting effects (positive or negative). The impact can be felt by them for the rest of their lives. One statement, one experience (whether we realize it or not) can make all the difference in the life and future of a child. Too often I have seen children exclusively blamed for their negative behaviors without adults taking the time to understand what is truly going on or why. Children, in many ways, are like flowers; they are delicate creatures whose environment primarily determines whether they grow healthy and strong or wither away and die.

It's important to understand that, with the exception of children who are born with mental health challenges, adults are responsible for the seeds we plant within our youth. We play a significant role in who children ultimately become. If we neglect them or damage their minds, bodies, or souls, society will be forced to deal with major consequences down the road.

Before we dive any further into the topic of children and therapy, it is necessary to state that neither this book nor this section is meant to be a parenting handbook. There is an abundance of books and resources available that explore the many complexities of parenting children. Some books have wonderful interventions, while others dive deeper into concepts, philosophies, and things to consider when trying to help raise emotionally healthy kids. Therefore, please understand that this chapter is simply an accumulation of the many observations I've made and the lessons I've learned working with children, adolescents, and their families in therapy.

TAKING A CHILD OR ADOLESCENT
TO THERAPY

As you can imagine, there are a variety of reasons why a parent may decide to take a child to receive mental health treatment. The main reason, of course, is because parents love their children and want to help them in any and every way possible. It's also likely the result of an adult seeing behaviors that are very concerning and possibly even harmful to their child or others. Some parents decide to bring their child to therapy because of the recommendations of others, such as teachers, family members, or friends. And then, although not as common, there are times when a young person tells their parents that they want to speak to someone, like a therapist. I am a firm believer that if a child or teenager specifically requests to see a clinician, it is in everyone's best interests to make sure that it happens.

When a child is brought to therapy, some parents expect that I will, within a few sessions, simply "fix" them. Meanwhile, they take on a more passive role and rarely participate in the overall treatment or therapy sessions. Now I'm not saying that a significant amount of therapeutic progress can't be made in a short period of time; however, I do not have a *magic wand*— although there have been plenty of times when I wish I did. The bottom line is that it is usually in the best interest of the child that the parent (or parents) and I work together.

The guardian (be it the mother, father, or primary caregiver) plays an important part in their child's treatment. We should be working collaboratively as a team. This does not necessarily mean that they will or should be a part of all or even most of the sessions, especially if they are the source of the problem. However, they should expect to be involved at some level, usually at the therapist's discretion. At the very least, I find it helpful when the parents of my child clients find some time to speak privately with me either immediately before or after a session. This can happen face-to-face or during a scheduled phone call.

CHILDREN IN THERAPY VERSUS TEENS IN THERAPY

As one would imagine, there are significant differences between a child being in therapy and an adolescent being in therapy.

Many children (usually twelve and under) are okay with going to treatment, especially if it is explained in a way that they can understand in order to reduce any fears or anxiety. This can be done by the parent or the clinician, but it's better if both participate in this discussion. Kids tend to be very cautious with new experiences, and some might not understand why they're in the office with this stranger in the first place. I usually try to ascertain why they think their parent brought them to me. This gives me a chance to learn how they see their situation and themselves, and what may be the best way to help them. This initial meeting also gives me a chance to observe how the child communicates, in addition to their character or personality traits, which will hopefully assist me with creating the therapeutic bond. If for some reason they are not sure why they're meeting with me, I try to communicate the concerns that their parent has for them in language that they can understand. I often tell the child how I want to help them become the best version of themselves. Ultimately, they are here because their parents love them very much, so much so that they want to do whatever they can to make sure they're happy and healthy.

When I learn that my new client is a teenager, however, I can't help but think of the line from *Forrest Gump* (with a slight modification): *teenagers* are like a box of chocolates; you never know what you're gonna get. In my experience, unless the adolescent has requested therapy, they are either very apprehensive about being in the session, would prefer not to be there, or flat-out don't believe they need therapy. If the teenager is not comfortable with or does not want to be in treatment, I try to respect their opinion while also attempting to understand how they see themselves and whether they see that what their parent is describing is an actual issue. I find it easier to explore this with my adolescent client in depth once I am alone with them (which usually happens after I've gone over confidentiality and its limitations). Once I am able to gain the teen's trust (as demonstrated by their overall comfort with speaking to me), we can then begin addressing what the challenges are. Many times teenagers have expressed gratitude for how they now have someone with whom they can share their thoughts or issues, and who will listen to them without judgment, criticism, or consequences.

One of the things I emphasize to parents when they bring their child or teenager to therapy is the importance of a healthy therapeutic relationship between their child and me. From the very first session, I always communicate to the parents that building rapport (as long as I know their child is safe physically and emotionally) is my first priority. I will ultimately get to whatever the issues are, but it is extremely difficult to address them if their child does not feel a positive connection with me.

Oh, the Places I've Been and the Kids I've Worked With

I spent a significant amount of my earlier years as a mental health professional working exclusively with children and their families. My first paid job after receiving my master's degree in psychology was working with teenagers in group homes. From there, I transitioned to the day-treatment program I mentioned earlier in this chapter, where children were brought to the facility after school. It was here where I gained my first experiences with restraining out-of-control kids whose behaviors, on occasion, would become so escalated that they were at risk of hurting someone (another child, a staff member, or possibly themselves). Years later, I found myself doing in-home therapy where I drove to various homes across Atlanta and surrounding cities in order to provide treatment.

One of the most challenging places I worked, where children were my primary clients, was at a residential treatment facility. This is the highest level of care a child or teenager can receive to address major behavioral or mental health problems. They would go to school and live on the grounds in small dorm-like buildings. They were fed three meals a day, and those who needed it were given medications daily. The facility was gated, with high fences and plenty of locks requiring keys to get in and out of most areas throughout the campus. This was basically the last stop for young people struggling with severe emotional health issues.

Unfortunately, these kids were considered extremely unsafe in their homes or at risk of hurting themselves or others. It's sad to say, but many of them were victims of abuse; some had experienced physical abuse, and many were victims of sexual abuse. It wasn't uncommon for them to have experienced both. A few of the young victims of sexual abuse became predators themselves and would have to be monitored very closely given the risk of them being sexually inappropriate with other kids in the facility.

Many of the children in this treatment center lacked the skills to effectively manage their feelings, especially when it came to controlling their anger. For this reason, every unit had what we called "time-out rooms," where individuals were required to stay until they de-escalated and were safe to be around others. The children and teenagers were typically there for months, and in some cases well over a year. We always hoped that parents would visit, and we encouraged them to, especially on weekends and holidays. The facility consisted of full-time nurses, a psychiatrist, clinicians, numerous support staff, aides, and teachers.

Being a part of the staff presented so many challenges— too many to get into in this book. However, I will say that while working in that residential treatment facility, I was sure of a few things: I would be involved in physically restraining an angry, volatile resident (probably ending up being hit or kicked). My patience level would be pushed to the max. I would receive plenty of practice with managing my own emotions (especially anger). And I would hear stories about the children's lives that would break my heart. It could be very disturbing to learn about the tragic and occasional mind-boggling abuse and destructive treatment that these kids experienced. Unfortunately, this speaks to the damage that can be done to a child by an adult who likely has their own mental health issues.

WHY ARE CHILDREN AND TEENS BROUGHT TO THERAPY?

As a clinician who has worked with children and teenagers for more than twenty years, I've seen a variety of reasons why a parent or guardian may seek treatment for their child. I will list many of them in this section, but some of the most common reasons are very similar to the reasons adults go to therapy: They are struggling with some aspect of their life. They're having difficulty managing their emotions, especially those associated with depression, anxiety, or both.

Some parents may not want to hear this, but adults play a major role in why so many of our youth feel so stressed, anxious, and depressed. Some parents contribute to their children's issues by, for example, not being aware of how their actions or inactions are negatively impacting their child. Perhaps as parents or guardians, they haven't taken the time to truly understand what their children's struggles are. After getting to know some of my clients, I have found myself wondering if some parents even know their child, and if they do, how well. Maybe the child does not feel loved. And who knows, maybe they aren't loved.

The Pressures Placed on Kids

There are a multitude of messages that are said or implied by parents and society that make it extremely difficult for a young person to manage what's going on in their life. I'm specifically referring to parents and a society that place greater and greater expectations on our youth. So often youth are being told by adults *what* they *should* be doing, *how* they *should* be doing it, *how* they *should feel* about something, *how* they *should* be performing, and what organizations or activities they *should* be a part of.

I'm not saying there should not be expectations; however, I am saying that if there are too many expectations (some of which may be unrealistic for a specific child), the pressure the child feels may lead to unintended consequences (stress, anxiety, depression).

There are times when teachers, other adults, or those in the media will catastrophize by saying that if children don't do such and such activities or make the right choices, their lives will be doomed forever. So many of my adolescent clients have been consumed with these thoughts, such as the belief that they must get into a certain college or else they will be failures.

For some teenagers, the academic pressures they experience in high school are so daunting that they just assume college will be even more difficult and therefore do not even consider higher education to be an option.

Then there is the increasing number of adolescent clients who are both driven and stressed with the belief that they must be wealthy (a millionaire or billionaire) or achieve something amazing ASAP. There is nothing wrong with having lofty goals—I support any and everyone's desire to dream big— however, some young adults have not thought about creating an actual plan for success, nor do they have an understating of the work and or sacrifice that will be required for them to accomplish their goals. Once a young person, especially a teen, feels overwhelmed as they strive to achieve certain objectives, they increasingly run the risk of struggling to manage possible disappointments and frustrations.

Adults must remember that kids are still growing and developing. They are going through both physical and cognitive changes every day. They're trying to adjust to their changing bodies and their evolving ways of thinking (about themselves, their lives, and the world). Many of them are trying to figure out who they are while also trying to fit in and have meaningful relationships with their peers. Just like adults, kids have their own struggles and experiences that parents may be completely unaware of.

I'll never forget the time my classmates and I were on our all-day eighth-grade-graduation trip, and I ended up being horribly embarrassed in front of my classmates. On the trip we were fortunate enough to ride in one of those nice luxury buses with air conditioning and comfortable seats, unlike the typical yellow school buses some of us rode on. I was sitting near the front with a group of what I would call the "regular kids." Unexpectedly, one of the "cool kids" came from the back and informed me that "Victoria" (not her real name; no need to make anyone feel guilty), the girl I adored and had a two-year crush on, wanted me to come to the back and join her, along with the other popular kids. Everyone, including Victoria, knew that I had always been crazy about her. Could this be the day she would reciprocate my feelings in a way that the whole world would know?

Unfortunately, my initial excitement came to a disappointing and abrupt conclusion. After eagerly getting up from my seat and going to the rear of the bus, I quickly realized that it wasn't to be the fairy tale I was hoping for. Victoria immediately launched into a series of jokes as she began teasing me (in front of everyone seated back there) about my off-brand Sears blue jeans. She and the rest of the cool kids erupted in laughter. While continuing to be the source of their amusement, I lowered my head, slowly turned around, and returned to my seat in the front area of the bus.

When it came to my clothes, I had no choice but to settle for what my mother could afford. She worked as a short-order cook and stretched her money as far as she could to take care of my sister and me. That meant familiar, high-quality, name-brand clothing was out of the question. She got us the most affordable and sometimes not the best quality clothing she could find. I didn't have a problem with the clothing I wore; I simply didn't spend much time thinking about it. My peers, however, didn't hesitate to let their thoughts about my attire be known. As you can imagine, it made me feel inadequate and sad and was definitely a punch to my self-esteem. This is just one small example of the challenges that a young person may experience that cause mental or emotional stress in their everyday life and that a parent will never know anything about.

Below is a list of the more common situations and behaviors I've seen with my young clients:

- Lack of motivation
- ADHD or its symptoms
- Problems with being defiant/oppositional

- Challenges with social skills or interacting with others
- Thoughts of or attempts at suicide
- Poor decision-making skills
- Frequent arguments
- Low self-esteem or feelings of inadequacy and insecurity
- Aggression (verbal or physical)
- Grief and loss
- Self-injurious behaviors (cutting, picking skin, pulling out hair)
- Substance use or abuse/addiction (drugs, alcohol, pornography)
- Frequent isolation
- Gender-identity struggles
- Depression
- Trauma
- Difficulty controlling anger
- Academic challenges or low or failing grades
- Anxiety
- Difficulties with life transitions/change
- The effects of abuse (physical or sexual)
- Loneliness or neglect
- Behavioral issues in school (negative attention-seeking behaviors, being disruptive)
- Challenges associated with being on the autism spectrum
- Feeling or being pressured by adults
- Placing pressure or stress on themselves

In many cases more than one of the above is present. Of course, other issues can be added to this list, but once again, these are the ones I have encountered most often.

I should also point out that the above-mentioned issues

can be experienced by adults as well; however, they are even more concerning or potentially damaging when a teen or pre-teen is trying to deal with them. When adolescents are struggling with these issues, it can be both intense and severe. As a result, many of these situations should be addressed as soon as possible.

MY ADOLESCENT INSECURITIES

Because the teenage years can be such a turbulent period, I think it is important to try to understand what is taking place in the mind of an adolescent. I have often told people, "You couldn't pay me enough to relive my high school days." When I reflect on that part of my life, there were definitely some good times and wonderful friendships. However, when I was a teen, I was constantly struggling with one thing or another. Of course, I was the typical adolescent trying to fit in with my peers while trying to figure life and myself out. I often felt invisible, despite having some pretty good friends, and I never felt special. Like so many people, I compared myself to others—never a wise decision, especially when you're young.

I wanted a girlfriend desperately, but no one at my school seemed to be interested in me—until my senior year, when I finally got my first official girlfriend. (FYI, it lasted three months.) I'm not saying girls didn't *like* me, because they did, but only as a friend. I frequently heard things like "You're like a brother to me." While I was banished to the "friend zone," they would tell me their problems, which primarily consisted of relationship struggles with boys who weren't treating them well. Oh, how I would be envious of the guys who had girlfriends or girls that liked them.

Girls weren't the only issue for me during high school. I struggled academically, especially in math and science classes.

I found it difficult to stay on top of all my assignments, which was primarily due to my not being organized and not knowing how to study. I was also in a program where I was forced to take all honors classes and then multiple AP classes during my senior year.

So there I was, not feeling good enough for girls to like me, struggling with my classes, arguing with my mother frequently, with no positive male role model in sight. But the most frustrating and disappointing aspect of high school was not being able to play football. You see, it was my dream to play high school football (then hopefully college and maybe even the pros) since I was a little boy. Unfortunately, I experienced a significant knee injury during my junior year that ultimately required major surgery, which I did not have until I was out of college. I did get to play my sophomore year but didn't get the true experience I hoped for because I was forced to play a position I didn't want. The emotional pain I experienced when a doctor told me that my high-school-football-playing days were over tore my heart apart. I try not to think about it much, but even now, I still feel the pain of disappointment, especially when I believed I had the ability to be a really great player.

Just like me, you likely have your own unforgettable teenage dramas and disappointments that made your earlier years mentally and emotionally challenging. Today, whether it's your children or someone else's, they, too, are trying to manage the stress and challenges in their world, often things that they have very little control over.

UNDERSTANDING WHAT TEENAGERS ARE DEALING WITH

As a therapist who has worked with a number of adolescents, I've been able to gain a better understanding of their motivations and issues. I have also seen things in their lives that remind me of my younger days—the commonalities many of us experienced that we seem to have forgotten now that we're adults. Let's identify some traits common to high schoolers. See if you recognize any of these in your own child or a teen you know, or if any take you back to your youth:

- The feelings and emotions of a teenager can be intense. Adults often accuse them of being "overly dramatic," which is understandable if we stop and think about it. What's become quite evident to me is that a lot of the feelings of adolescents are heightened, if not exaggerated (at least from an adult's perspective). I often say when it comes to teenagers, all of their emotions are "extra." When an adolescent is angry, it's often so unnecessarily over-the-top that you have to hope nothing gets broken or a younger sibling is not about to get hurt. When a teen is happy, they are some of the goofiest people to be around. When they are sad, it's as if the world itself has stopped and as if *no one* in the history of mankind has ever felt the pain that they're experiencing. This transitional period of *not quite being an adult but also not wanting to be treated like a child* is often very challenging (if not confusing) for both parents and teens.
- Many teenagers are often wrapped in a blanket of insecurities. They struggle with feeling like they are not enough. Their minds are filled with questions, doubt, and uncertainty: "Am I physically attractive?" "Do I have the right clothes?" "Am I liked by my friends?" "Am I cool?" "What is my future going to look like?" "Will I be successful?"

"Do I have true friends?" "Will I find love?" "Am I lovable?" "Am I capable of getting good grades?"

- They undergo hormonal changes. Quite a bit of the literature points to how the sex hormones estrogen and testosterone impact an adolescent's brain, causing them to be moodier.[1] In addition, other changes going on in the brain appear to affect their ability to manage stress, anxiety, and depression, and to make healthy choices. Their brains are still growing, and much of the information seems to indicate that the human brain is still developing until the early twenties, particularly in the frontal lobe where reasoning, judgment, and impulse control are located.[2]

- Teens want to feel like they fit in. As humans, we all have a natural desire to be a part of a community, to be connected to something bigger than ourselves. We are social creatures; therefore most of us tend to want to be around others. When that doesn't happen, we feel isolated and alone, a state we typically try to avoid. Many people spend a significant portion of their lives trying to find "their people" or "their tribe," a place where they feel comfortable, accepted, and even valued. This is a reason why some teenagers join sports teams and social clubs, while others join street gangs.

- Adolescents often are in conflict with their parents or parental figures. (I know I was, and I wouldn't be surprised if you were as well.) This is sometimes due to teens asserting themselves more (or at least trying to do so) as they attempt to create some degree of independence. Remember, although they are not yet fully adults with adult responsibilities, they typically no

longer want to be treated like or spoken to as
young children.

- Teenagers want to be accepted for the way they
are. Adolescents tend to struggle with comments
from others, especially if they feel they are being
criticized. They are therefore vulnerable to being
overcome with insecurities and self-doubt. They
typically have not yet learned how to prevent the
words of others from emotionally triggering or
negatively impacting them. This is made even
more difficult when so many times adults (be it
parents, teachers, or even other family members)
do a poor job of trying to address teens' concerns.

- For adolescents, peer pressure is real and can
make life very challenging. Often peer pressure
is the result of teenagers wanting to fit in; therefore they may go along with the group (even if
this means doing something that is potentially
dangerous, immoral, or illegal). Peer pressure can
come in many forms, including being teased or
being made to feel guilty for doing, or not doing,
something.

- The role of social media in their lives is more
significant than we can imagine. I'm extremely
grateful that I grew up when the internet didn't
exist. I believe that technology, screens, and
social media are simultaneously society's greatest
blessing *and* a curse. This definitely appears to be
true for adolescents. Not only are many of them
addicted to their screens, but they are also more
vulnerable to this influence. Unfortunately, for
some, social media provides them with a way to
escape personal issues, whereas others get sucked
in to comparing themselves (their lives, how they

look, and what they have) to people who are likely
presenting an image that is not real or true.

As if navigating all this isn't enough, teens can experience
conflicts within their homes, be victims of abuse, and feel the
impact of financial struggles, addiction, and/or mental health
issues in the family. When we consider all the things that an
adolescent is likely to endure, it becomes quite evident how
challenging this period of their life can be. To further com-
plicate matters, many have few or no coping strategies to deal
with their problems, nor do they have an adult they feel they
can turn to for help. As a result, they may try to manage things
in their own way (or take the advice of their peers, which may
not be a great idea) and engage in activities they believe will
help them but instead make matters even worse.

BEGINNING TREATMENT WITH
CHILDREN AND ADOLESCENTS

When I first meet with a new young client, I divide the session
into three parts. First, I like to meet with the parents privately
in order to allow them to freely share their concerns about
their child. I've learned in the past that if the child or teen is
present when the parents are describing their issues, the child
or teen may feel very uncomfortable (and I may as well) or criticized. Who wants to sit next to their parents as they divulge
what is likely very personal information to a total stranger, especially when what's disclosed is not only uncomfortable but
also downright embarrassing?

Next, I have the young person join us. At this time, my
goals include observing the family's interactions with one another as well as their body language. I ask my young client if
they know why their parents have brought them to meet me,

and then review with them confidentiality and its limitations. I want the teen or child (and the parents) to understand that there will be things discussed that will stay between the teen or child and myself. Despite my desire to maintain this level of confidentiality, there are also things I won't keep private, such as any type of abuse or neglect and attempts or thoughts of suicide. I also make it clear that things may have to be disclosed if I am subpoenaed, and it's also possible that I may discuss their issues with other clinicians working in my office.

For the final portion of the initial session, I usually prefer it to just be the client and me. It's extremely important to me to begin building the therapeutic relationship as soon as possible. As a matter of fact, I believe that if a young client doesn't feel comfortable and safe with me, it will be very difficult to achieve the therapeutic goals or resolve the issues that brought them to therapy. Establishing a healthy relationship is so important that I try to make sure the parents understand that, aside from prioritizing their overall safety, developing a comfortable connection with their child is my first goal. I am not sure how other clinicians work with younger clients, but this is my method and it has been successful for me during my twenty years of being a mental health professional.

How long does it take for the therapeutic relationship to get to a good, stable place? It depends. Every child is different. I will say that for younger clients, if I'm able to connect with them either through an area of interest or through play activities, the process typically may only take a couple of sessions. Teens, however, tend to be a little bit more suspicious and cautious. Therefore it can be unclear how long it will take for me to get to know them while also gaining their trust. A lot of teenagers typically either don't want to be in therapy or don't believe they need to be, so building this relationship requires creativity, empathy (while demonstrating interest in their lives), and definitely patience.

THE VALUE OF FOSTERING A HEALTHY RELATIONSHIP BETWEEN PARENT AND CHILD

It's hard for me to imagine any relationship as important as the one between a parent and their child. The bond between them, or the lack thereof, can play a significant role in how that young person grows up, who they eventually become, and how they will impact society and the world. This may be surprising to hear, but I have come across parents who struggle with forming, or are completely unable to form, a healthy emotional connection with their child. Typically these parents or guardians may not know how to connect but they do know how to correct or criticize their children when they've done "wrong." The parent will communicate their expectations for their kids, but I hope they're also able to examine how often they criticize their children compared to how often they praise or encourage them.

Many parents are also really good at pushing their children to perform at high levels (sometimes leading to stress and anxiety within the child). We should, of course, encourage them to be the best they possibly can be; however, I also believe that too much of a good thing can be bad. Pushing the child could result in the child becoming emotionally distant, and thus damage the relationship.

It is important for parents to know the strengths, weaknesses, likes, and dislikes of their children. I wish I saw more parents who are committed to knowing who their kids are and willing to learn what's in their hearts and minds. It's not uncommon for my teen or preteen clients to tell me their parents don't know who they are and don't spend quality one-on-one time with them. For most relationships to grow, whether with a friend, a partner, or a child, individuals must make the effort to get to know and understand one another. Even the relationship between a dog and its owner is strengthened by spending quality time together.

Most of my younger clients share things with me that they don't feel comfortable sharing with their parents. Some believe their parents would not understand, will judge them, or will minimize their thoughts and feelings. I've had clients who excitedly shared their interests with me, and when I've asked if they've also disclosed this to their parents, they say, "They don't really care," or "They don't understand why I like _____," (fill in the blank) or "They're always busy." There is a lot of value in a parent sharing their child's interests in order to strengthen the relationship between them.

The Ideal Relationship Between Children and Parents

In an ideal situation, the relationship between an adult and a young person would have a healthy balance of nurturing and instruction given to the child. This can be done by giving them encouragement when necessary and correcting them when they've made choices that are not in their best interest. Children would be raised in environments where they feel heard, seen, and understood. They would grow up in homes where they learned important values required to produce an adult of strong character. In an ideal world, they would also develop high self-esteem and learn the values of being kind, resilient, and respectful of others. And finally, if not most importantly, they would observe, learn about, and experience love—both receiving and giving it—through the interactions between themselves and their parents and other family members. Of course, there are many other positive seeds that should be planted in youth, but if these foundational principles are present, I believe there is a greater chance of them growing up to become people who can help this world become a better place for us all.

Unfortunately, we don't live in an ideal world, and everyone is not equipped with the skills or experience needed to have a healthy and nurturing relationship with their children. Some parents never heal their own wounds from growing up and therefore pass them on to their kids. Some people who become parents may not have wanted to do so. If we get totally honest, we should acknowledge the fact that not everyone should be a parent, just as not everyone should be married, go to college, or own a home. Everything isn't for everybody.

When parents are unable (or even unwilling) to invest the time, energy, nurturing, and love into their relationship with their children, there can be devastating consequences. When a healthy connection is not present, children can struggle with feeling bad about themselves or develop low self-esteem. They may end up with poor coping skills and struggle to deal with emotions like sadness and anger. Parents who haven't provided what children need make it more difficult for their children to build the necessary resiliency to push through life's challenges.

If a child lacks the support and love they need, there is a greater chance they will grow up lacking the skills to form healthy relationships as adults. I have seen multiple instances when a dysfunctional upbringing has led to a client (or friend) becoming repeatedly involved in relationships that are supposed to be loving yet are anything but that. Instead, they find themselves in situations that are harmful physically, mentally, emotionally, or even spiritually. Hopefully, if they do find themselves in these "situationships," they are able to acknowledge the role that their upbringing (including the wounds that may have been produced during that time) may have played and decide to seek help, professional or otherwise. If they don't, they may become parents themselves and continue the cycle of not meeting the emotional needs of their children.

Our Responsibilities to Our Youth

Adults are responsible for the youth and future generations, even if they are not parents. Whether you're a teacher, coach, counselor, accountant, entrepreneur, city worker, government employee, janitor, aunt, uncle, or even a neighbor, I believe you should do what you can to help young people become the best people they can be. Most parents feel that when it comes to taking care of children, theirs are the main priority; therefore they don't have the time, energy, or desire to address the needs of someone else's kids. Undoubtedly, there's a lot of truth in that statement, and I respect and understand that viewpoint. Your children should be your priority, especially given how difficult the job of being a parent can be. However, please realize that if you choose to completely ignore the well-being and mental health of other young people, their issues may ultimately be forced upon you, your community, and possibly even your child.

We all play a part in what happens to future generations, whether you're a parent or not, through our actions, our words, and the morals and values we pass on (or don't pass on) to the young. Yes, in a perfect world every parent would develop compassion, a work ethic, resiliency, discernment, and intelligence in their kids. In a perfect world, parents, guardians, and adults in general would give kids far more praise than criticism. However, we know this is not always the case. I think as adults we should heed the African proverb "It takes a village to raise a child." I have heard this many times but often wonder if we really believe it. If we believe there is truth in this statement, are we willing to be active participants in the village and not just spectators who complain? Are we going to be "that adult" from an older generation who generalizes and makes stereotypical comments like "Kids today are lazy, disrespectful, materialistic, shallow, superficial, sensitive"?

I believe we all should contribute to helping the young people in our lives understand the values of working hard, caring for others, developing patience, building resiliency, and judging people by their character and not by their appearance, race, religion, socioeconomic status, sex, gender, or gender preference.

As Adults, Let's Take More Responsibility

Many of the things we complain about as they relate to children and teens are our fault. We are the adults after all, so how can we not assume some responsibility for how younger generations turn out? Many adults say they feel younger generations are entitled, spoiled, or soft, but who gave them everything they asked for? Adults did. We know many kids spend a lot of time on screens, whether it's their cell phone or a video game, but they didn't invent those things. Adults did. We are the ones who purchased those items and then allowed our kids to spend too much time using them. I've heard adults complain about drug use among teenagers, but who grows, imports, and sells the drugs?

I've talked about the violence so often reported in the news, but who builds and sells the guns, who manufactures the bullets, who makes the television shows and the films that contain an inordinate number of acts of violence? Who gives recording contracts to singers and rap artists whose lyrics often contain images of aggression (if not outright violence) or who engage in a host of destructive behaviors?

I find it extremely interesting that there are those in our society who believe they are taking care of our kids by banning books they think will negatively impact them, yet seem to be okay with kids' minds being flooded with images of violence, sex, materialism, divisiveness, and greed from a variety of sources. Are our children raising themselves, or are the adults mishandling their God-given calling?

I have met with so many parents who seem to expect their children to always make the right choices, while ignoring their own hypocritical behaviors, which may include an unwillingness to work on their own personal issues. Some adults, whether they are parents are not, are poor role models due to their inability to teach or nurture healthy relationships. These adults may never have been exposed to positive, healthy parenting and lack this knowledge or, in extreme cases, are not interested in supporting and loving their child. If an adult lacks the skills to be a "good" parent, is it realistic to expect their child to grow up and become an incredibly well-rounded, successful individual who is both emotionally and mentally healthy? I don't think so.

DISCIPLINE AND PUNISHMENT

The stress of exposure to frequent yelling alone may be as detrimental to a child's health as physical punishment.

—Kelli Harding, MD, MP

As one would imagine, there are many different interventions and parenting styles that adults may use when they feel their child needs to be disciplined. Methods parents choose to punish children are usually based on how the parents were punished, the age of the parents, the age of the children, the parents' thoughts about punishment, and the culture in which the parents identify.

Regardless of one's thoughts or methods when it comes to discipline, there are times when children must learn the relationship between actions and consequences. Kids must learn that if Mom says, "Don't touch the stove! It's hot!" and they do it anyway, it is likely the outcome won't be good. Punishing the child becomes a way to try to correct possible negative or inappropriate behaviors in the hopes that they do not occur again, with the expectation that they learn how to make the best choices they possibly can now and for the rest of their life.

Children are going to make mistakes, and that includes doing things they probably shouldn't as well as not doing things they probably should. Sometimes they will make the same mistakes over and over. I have heard from countless parents how aggravating this can be. I've also worked with parents who have unrealistic expectations for their children to do the right thing *all the time* or learn a lesson immediately. Parenting is a difficult task that requires a ton of patience, understanding, forgiveness, and maybe even some prayer (for both the parent and child). When children require correction, it's important to identify the most effective ways that do not cause irreparable mental, emotional, or physical harm.

The types of punishments a parent decides to use on their kids are significant and can yield positive or possibly negative effects. I believe whether and how a child is punished should depend on a variety of factors, including, but not limited to, what the child has done, how often the behavior has occurred, their age, their emotional or psychological development, the child's history (including any history of abuse or trauma), physical/mental disabilities, the parent, and what resources are available to possibly help the family. Even the individual personality of the child should be considered when trying to decide how to teach them important lessons.

Spare the Rod, Spoil the Child?

I was raised by a single African American mother from a tiny rural Mississippi town. Many parents from that area and time period tended to believe in the proverb "Spare the rod, spoil the child." If you are unfamiliar with this, it's inspired by Proverbs 13:24: "He who spares the rod hates his son. But he who loves him disciplines him promptly" (NKJV). Many people have interpreted this to mean that not only are they justified in using corporal punishment (when adults deliberately inflict physical pain on a child to correct or eliminate negative behaviors), they believe they *should* use it. This typically involved being struck multiple times with an open hand, a switch (a branch from a bush or tree), or, if the child was older, a belt, paddle, piece of wood, shoe, or even an extension cord—whatever was within arm's reach of the parent. And my mother was apparently a true believer in this method of punishment.

In the seventies when I was growing up, we did not have the same laws to protect children from being abused that exist today. As a matter of fact, from what I've been able to ascertain, federal legislation to protect children didn't come online until the mid to late seventies. Therefore many parents did pretty much whatever they felt needed to be done in order to punish or send a strong message to their children. From first through fourth grade, I attended a Catholic school. Our teachers were nuns and were actually allowed to hit us (multiple times) with their paddles (at my school this usually meant being struck on the palms of our hands).

I feel very confident in saying that the ways in which children were often punished during that period would be classified as child abuse today, especially in my case where there were often bruises on my body when my mother chose an extension cord as her way of teaching me a lesson. There were times when I questioned whether my mother loved me as I was being administered my punishments. At that age, I figured there was no way a parent could love their child and cause the pain that I was experiencing.

Despite that what happened to me would be considered abuse today, looking back as an adult I realize she was trying to raise me the best way she knew how. She was raising me the way she and her siblings were raised, as well as the way others in her community were raised during that time. I believe she thought she was doing that "for my own good." She wanted me to be a "good boy" and ultimately grow up to be an obedient, responsible adult. To be quite frank with you, I think she was successful in doing that. I do not believe I have unresolved childhood trauma or wounds as a result of how she chose to teach me consequences.

Although I'm extremely confident that I was not negatively impacted by the way my mother chose to punish me, I'm sure there are those who were. Please know that I am in no way advocating that children should be hit as a way of punishing them. I believe there is more than one way of doing anything, and there are definitely other ways to provide consequences to a child without having to strike them. Plus, we now have local agencies and laws in place to protect children if it is believed that a parent, guardian, or other adult is physically hurting them. If someone thinks or sees evidence that a child has been or is being abused, they can and should file a report with the proper authorities, and an investigation is likely to follow, possibly resulting in the child being removed from their home and placed with other family members or in a foster home.

When a parent or guardian has decided that punishment is necessary to correct or eliminate inappropriate behaviors, it is important to try to understand why the child has done what they've done (or not done). Perhaps the child is dealing with some unknown external stressors—a difficult teacher, bullies, social exclusion at school, and so on. Perhaps someone has been abusing or hurting them and no one is aware. Maybe the child's negative behaviors are because they are struggling with changes within their home or the family. Perhaps they're feeling unloved or not supported by their parents. Then there is also the possibility that a child or adolescent is dealing with some previously undiagnosed mental health or physical issue.

The bottom line here is that there are likely reasons behind their inappropriate behaviors, and punishing them without trying to find out what these reasons are is counterproductive and will not solve the true problem.

Using corporal punishment can change or eliminate negative behaviors in a child, but is it the right thing to do? When delivering consequences, parents and guardians have a variety of options to consider.

Corporal punishment is an extreme option, and there are times when it may also be questionable if not outright inappropriate. If the parent of a client I'm working with believes that some degree of physical force is necessary to correct certain behaviors, I have very limited say in the matter. However, please be aware that using this form of discipline, especially when upset or angry, is often how children end up being physically abused.

There are a variety of other ways to provide consequences to children that do not include laying hands on or striking them. Depending on the circumstances, the child, the child's age, and the parent, other ways may be more effective. Some commonly used interventions for teens include placing restrictions or taking away privileges (e.g., not being able to drive their car or use their cell phone, loss of extracurricular activities). Other methods to consider for both teens and younger children are the addition of chores or other responsibilities (especially tasks that young people would rather avoid), praise or compliments for doing the correct thing, time-outs (primarily with younger children), restrictions on spending time with friends or attending events, incentives and rewards, writing assignments about their feelings and the inappropriateness of their actions, and a host of other interventions.

When I was young and hadn't done my chores, my mother

had the perfect way to encourage me to handle my responsibilities. She wouldn't allow me to go outside and play. When I was growing up, nothing felt as torturous as knowing your friends were outside playing while you were imprisoned within your own home. I remember so many times when my friends came to my house, rang the doorbell, and asked, "Can Frank come out to play?" only to hear my mom tell them, "No, because he didn't do his chores!" Clearly a different time and a different generation. Nowadays, children typically *don't* want to go outside, may have to be forced to do so, and would much rather be indoors on their devices for hours on end.

Finally, I don't want to ignore the damage that can be inflicted upon a child as a result of the words spoken by their parents, guardians, other adult family members, teachers, and influential people in the child's life (especially if these words are yelled, are demeaning, destroy the child's self-esteem, are hurtful, are unnecessarily critical or judgmental, are profanity-laced, cause them to experience anxiety/depression, or are outright mean). I realize that sometimes adults yell at children as a result of being frustrated and angry; however, what is said and how it is said can have a long-lasting effect and be more damaging than the loss of privileges, or even corporal punishment. Someone is reading this who knows exactly what I mean because they experienced the negative effects of verbal abuse when they were young.

There is no single, magical way of disciplining children that is effective every time or with every child. This is why I strongly recommend that parents who are struggling with trying to get their children to behave, or are struggling with how to punish them, utilize the many resources that we have at our disposal. This could mean meeting with a clinician, finding a support group, taking parenting classes, reading the vast number of books that have been written about the subject, gaining insight from friends, and getting the support of other family members.

Raising children can be, and often is, an extremely challenging and demanding job. Parents get angry and frustrated with their kids, and kids get angry and frustrated with their parents. Just remember that there are no perfect children, no perfect parents, and no perfect families.

Entitlement

Today many believe that our youth are "spoiled." They think that children have been raised by parents who freely and repeatedly give them whatever it is they ask for. With this being the case, it is easy to see how a child becomes conditioned to expect things to go their way. Always catering to what a child wants, however, can lead to them developing what's often described as "a sense of entitlement." This is when they believe that they should always get what they want, when they want it, and how they want it—whatever *it* may be.

This sense of entitlement often emerges over a period of time as a result of parents simply trying to both show their love and please their child. After all, who doesn't want to see their children happy? There are also times when a parent wants to prevent their child from being disappointed or emotionally hurt. Many parents will do everything in their power to prevent their offspring from feeling hurt or their self-esteem from taking a hit. I see nothing wrong with parents trying to protect children, trying to make them happy, or doing what they believe is in the child's best interest. However, as I mentioned before, I also believe too much of a good thing can be bad.

RESILIENCY AND CHILDREN

Most of us have figured out by now that life can be difficult, full of challenges, and outright frustrating. However, most of us have also learned that regardless of our situation, it's extremely important to do our best to push through obstacles that come our way. In doing so, we demonstrate what it means to be *resilient*, something that I believe should start in childhood. Developing resiliency early ultimately prepares children for the many unexpected challenges that will come their way as adults.

As a therapist and an adjunct college instructor, I've become very concerned about the lack of resiliency demonstrated by the younger generations. The fact that many feel that kids and young adults today are "soft, coddled, and spoiled" is a subject that has been explored in articles, interviews, and discussions. I have witnessed instances in which children, teens, and young adults struggle with disappointment, finding it difficult to manage their emotions when something doesn't go the way they had hoped (whether it be a grade they wanted, an electronic device they had to have, a certain peer liking them, or a particular job they wanted).

Questioning Whether We Are Building Resilient Youth

I often find myself questioning whether adults, and society in general, truly understand the importance of building mental and emotional fortitude in the young. Are we considering the possibility that by being overprotective or overly accommodating, we are doing more harm than good? I wonder whether the emphasis should be on protecting children's emotions or on strengthening them for the future. Are we preparing our children for the realities of life without going overboard, stressing them out, and scaring them half to death? Are we helping them better understand the importance of getting back up after experiencing a setback? Maybe more attention should be given to the idea that adversity is often necessary for growth and that failure is not forever. On many occasions, failure is a learning experience and a prerequisite to success. I question whether the younger generations are being exposed to the value of knowing that there will be times when things are completely out of their control. In these moments, it's important to learn about acceptance and the need to be flexible to achieve a goal, or maybe create new goals altogether.

Appreciating Life's Challenges

Regardless of age, challenges will arise, but if we can focus on striving to be resilient while viewing challenges differently, life can become more manageable. I believe that some of the trials we all face can make life interesting, if not exciting. Hopefully, we also grow as a result. When we experience difficulties, I believe once we get past them, we'll have an opportunity to appreciate having grown through them. We typically value beautiful, sunny days even more because of the dark, rainy days. We can enjoy laughter so much more because we've cried. Many of us cherish quality time with others because we've also experienced the pain of being alone. But in the end, these are all things that are a part of life. Perhaps we should try to plant this mindset into the minds of our young.

It is my hope that parents, guardians, or adults who have children in their lives will help them to be like trees with deep, solid roots. Roots so strong that no matter what extreme weather conditions are present, no matter how intense the storms of life may be, they will remain firmly able to stand.

The Value of Saying No to Children

Telling a child no when it's appropriate presents a great opportunity for them to learn or be reminded about boundaries. When a child becomes accustomed to always getting what they want, it increases the likelihood of them taking for granted the things they do have.

When a young person is being told no for practical or important reasons, they are being presented with an opportunity for growth. I believe that when a child or teen is told no followed by an explanation, they are provided with an opportunity to work on coping skills, learn ways to manage feelings of disappointment, understand rules, accept boundaries, strengthen their resiliency, and prepare for life as an adult—a time in which they will undoubtedly be told no many times and in a variety of situations and settings, especially when things are out of their control.

When I was young, whenever I was told no, I always asked my mother, "But why?" She couldn't stand it when I did this. She rarely explained why and would ultimately get so upset at my repeated questioning that she would end the discussion by saying, "Because I said so!" I'm pretty sure she felt I was questioning her authority, but I promise you I was not. I simply wanted to understand the reason behind the decision. Someone is reading this who can totally relate to me as a child.

INTERVENTIONS AND TREATMENT

When it comes to working with children and teens, there is no one specific intervention that is guaranteed to help them deal with their mental, emotional, or behavioral challenges. Whatever issues they're experiencing, each child is different, and what works for one may not work for another—even though they may have similar situations or diagnoses.

The same is also true for medications considered as a form of treatment. All medications do not work for everyone. Taking a certain pill may relieve my headache, but it may do absolutely nothing to get rid of yours. Therefore it's important that I, as a mental health professional, gain as much information about the young client as I can in order to effectively help them. For me, this includes nailing down an accurate diagnosis, being aware of the young client's individual challenges and personal history, and being open-minded about different treatments. I also accept the fact that if one thing doesn't work, I still can consider other possibilities.

As a therapist working with adolescents and younger kids, I ultimately have to identify how to produce change by doing one or both of the following: first, finding the correct interventions to help with modifying their behaviors, and second, helping them see or think in more positive, healthy, productive, or beneficial ways.

However, if I had to identify one intervention that's been most helpful for my clients, it would be building a strong bond or connection with them. When they know they have someone they can talk to who is an attentive and caring listener, that alone can produce amazing results.

I remember, while I was working in the school system providing mental health treatment, several teachers praised me for the progress I had made with one of their students who happened to be my ten-year-old client. What's interesting is, at that point, he was still relatively new to me, and I really hadn't started implementing any specific activities, goals, or interventions. However, every week I still came to his school to meet with him. It became apparent that the individualized attention he was receiving from me, regardless of what we did during our meetings, was producing such a positive effect that it significantly reduced the negative behaviors he was displaying in his classroom.

Final Thoughts

Finally, when working with children, I think it is extremely valuable to use a holistic approach. For me this means not just ensuring their mental and emotional needs are met, but also exploring whether their physical needs are being met. Once I have a thorough understanding of the presenting problem, sooner or later I question the parents about their child's diet, sleep habits, water intake, and physical activity levels. I'm also likely to ask if they've had a thorough physical exam recently that includes assessment for vitamin deficiencies and insulin/blood sugar levels. I explore these things with parents because a child's emotional and mental well-being can be significantly impacted by poor health or health-related issues.

If you are a parent or guardian, please stay up to date with your child's annual physical exams; encourage your child to get proper rest, drink plenty of water, and reduce their sugar intake; and provide them with the healthiest foods possible. There's a plethora of accessible information out there about healthy living and lifestyle choices that can benefit both children and adults. I encourage talking to a dietitian or your primary care physician in order to ensure your child is the healthiest they possibly can be.

CHAPTER 7

Lessons Learned About Self-Care

*Yesterday I was clever so I wanted to change
   the world.*
Today I am wise so I'm changing myself.

—Rumi

I'd like you to take a moment and picture a healthy middle-aged woman walking alone along a desolate road. The path that she is on is nothing out of the ordinary. Parts of it are level, some areas have a slight incline, while other sections have a slight decline. In some locations there are rocks, branches, and other debris, while other parts are quite smooth and uncluttered.

As you continue visualizing this woman, you notice that she is carrying several boxes of various sizes and weights. She occasionally adjusts the parcels when they become too heavy or her arms become fatigued. As she continues down the path, the woman encounters other boxes that she's intent on picking up and adding to the ones she already has. After much thought and careful adjustment, this woman finds a way to pick up even more, despite being tired and overwhelmed, and is now clearly carrying too many.

She's moving slower and slower; her arms are continuing to get weaker and weaker as she walks hunched over, trying to continue carrying her load. She is physically and mentally exhausted, suffering, and yelling out in agony due to her immense discomfort. How much more of this can she take? Doesn't she know there is only so much she can do, and for only a certain amount of time?

This is a metaphor for what many of my clients and friends are doing as they take on too many tasks or set too many goals that ultimately cause them to feel overwhelmed and stressed. I feel confident in saying that there are times when many of us take on so much in our lives that it's to our own detriment. I'm guilty of doing this on more than one occasion. We take on tasks that may be very necessary and important while neglecting the fact that we may be doing too much for too long.

There are times when we would best be served by determining which boxes are most important to carry and which ones to put down, perhaps to pick up later or maybe never again. Maybe we are strong enough to carry the load. But even if that's true, we are not machines. From time to time, we all need rest, which may mean putting the boxes down, even if it's only for a short period. Once rested and rejuvenated, we can then resume down our path, carrying what we feel needs to be carried.

To me, this is the essence of why self-care is extremely important. I believe a good portion of self-care should include knowing oneself—our weaknesses, strengths, and boundaries (i.e., when to say no)—which allows us to successfully navigate the stressors in our lives.

I have found that more than half of my adult clients are struggling emotionally, and perhaps physically and spiritually, because they aren't successfully incorporating self-care into their lives. I have also learned that people simply do not take the time to regularly engage in activities that may provide them with temporary relief from their extensive to-do lists.

It's very common for women to place their spouses, children, jobs, and even friends before their own emotional and mental well-being. Don't get me wrong, I don't believe there's anything wrong with prioritizing your loved ones and your career. However, I also believe if you don't take care of yourself, if you don't nurture yourself, if you don't give yourself downtime, if you don't rest, then you run the risk of being unable to effectively take care of those things and people you love so much. Some clients are so committed to serving others that they feel guilty if they even attempt to take time out for themselves.

WHAT IS SELF-CARE?

I define self-care and self-care interventions as activities that focus on taking care of one's overall sense of well-being. In other words, doing things that make you feel good, at ease, and peaceful; provide a healthy break from the norm; and ultimately help with effectively managing the stressors of life. By focusing on taking care of your personal needs, you give yourself the opportunity to be renewed, to do your job better, and to take care of others. Self-care is where we find time to nurture our mind, our body, and our spirit. Self-care is caring for the self.

The Need for Self-Care

Thanks to movies, television programs, magazines, and social media, we've been led to believe that we need to have certain things and look a certain way in order to be valuable or significant. We've been led to think that only specific achievements define success. Attempting to measure up to what others believe we need to be can easily result in people feeling stressed, insecure, overwhelmed, anxious, and depressed, and for some this can cause physical issues such as ulcers, high blood pressure, or panic attacks.

For many, the stressors of life can become so overwhelming that they choose coping mechanisms that are potentially harmful or addictive. These behaviors can include overuse or abuse of alcohol and drugs, risky sexual practices, excessive shopping, eating disorders, self-injury (cutting, hair-pulling), and taking frustrations out on others verbally or physically. I've seen how trying to manage today's stressors and meet society's expectations can be too difficult for some as they cling to sanity.

We've allowed the world to pressure us to the point where we think that our lives have to be a certain way—or that we absolutely must have specific things in order to be happy, successful, or at peace—and anything short of that simply won't suffice. This can significantly affect our self-esteem and our ability to experience the joy of life, causing us to have more sadness and depression.

Expectations of Society

Before we continue, let's look at some typical expectations that many of us allow others to place on us, negatively impacting how we navigate the world around us:

- Having to agree with the ideas of your parents
- Feeling as if one has to get good grades in school in order to go to college (perhaps even a certain college) and then get a great job

- Being forced to believe in God or have certain religious or spiritual beliefs
- Being expected to get married
- Being expected to have children now or in the future
- Being told home ownership is a necessity
- Feeling that you are not successful unless you make a lot of money or achieve a certain socio-economic level
- Feeling you must attain a certain look to be considered attractive
- Being driven to compete and win at all costs
- Feeling irrelevant unless you become a person of importance, notoriety, or popularity
- Feeling you must be strong, both emotionally and physically
- Feeling you must dress a certain way (e.g., only wearing name-brand clothing) to be relevant
- Feeling you must drive a certain type of car
- Feeling you must be really great or talented at something, or become the best at something

When people are solely focused on living up to society's expectations, they are likely not being true to themselves. They may not know what it is they want out of their life, let alone how to obtain it. Then there are those who have some idea of what they want for themselves but lack the courage to do what they were meant to do or be the person they were meant to be. I believe it is extremely important to identify your true, authentic self and honor the person you are, or who you were meant to be. For some this may mean not trying to meet all the expectations that everyone else has for you.

WHY DON'T WE MAKE SELF-CARE A PRIORITY?

I believe the most important, and probably the most over-looked, relationship is the one we have with ourselves. As a therapist, I take the time to learn about the various relation-ships that a client has in their life. Eventually, I like to discover what they think about themselves. It is not uncommon for me to ask questions such as "Do you like yourself?" Or, further, "Do you love yourself?" You'd be surprised how many peo-ple struggle with these questions and respond, "I don't know. I'm not sure. I think so." More unfortunately, some say, "No, I don't love myself." Perhaps you are someone who's unsure how to answer these questions.

On many occasions, a client verbalizing that they don't like or love themselves is an indication that they are struggling to heal from past trauma. Unresolved pain can manifest in a variety of ways, including low self-esteem, depression, anxiety, or unhealthy or toxic behaviors (e.g., addictions). When people do not care enough about themselves, they may take it out on others by mistreating them. This mistreatment can take the form of verbal or physical abuse directed at partners, family, friends, or coworkers.

If we truly want to change our lives, we must begin with ourselves. My clients, and people in general, often find them-selves repeatedly experiencing the same hurts and disap-pointments. If this is the case for you, it is time to take some responsibility for your life.

I remember when I was living in my small studio apart-ment in Southern California and not liking the way my life was looking. I barely had enough money to pay my bills, I was often alone, and I lacked connection with others. Then one day it hit me: *Perhaps I am playing a major role in how my life is turning out right now.* I became convinced that I was responsible for my current situation, so I took an index card and wrote, "You are responsible for how your life is right now." Then I posted it on my desktop monitor. Every time I sat in front of my computer screen, I would read those words. It felt like I was being punched in the stomach because I knew I had the power to do things differently, or at least try. I knew that it was time to change the thoughts, actions, and beliefs that were holding me back from a more fulfilling life.

Whether we realize it or not, or choose to accept it or not, our outer world changes when our inner world changes. I try to help clients with understanding the value of knowing this as well as how even one small step toward positive transformation or healing matters. Hopefully they are then willing to take another small step, then another, and another. If this is done over time, progress will certainly be made. But having said that, please don't beat yourself up if you are unable, or find it difficult, to take those small steps. Try to avoid setting unrealistic expectations, and don't create a timeline for when something *must* be accomplished. Doing so only produces stress and opens the door to disappointment if you're unable to meet a deadline. Don't be so hard on yourself. A lot of things in this life take time to accomplish.

People thinking negatively about themselves serves no real purpose other than making them feel worse. This is why it is so important for people to forgive themselves and learn to like themselves, and ultimately to love themselves. So much of what we experience in life is about learning, healing, and growing through our challenges.

Making Excuses

> *I urge you to simply accept the fact that you'll never get it all done, and begin to live more fully in the only moment that you have—now!*

> —Wayne Dyer

I have heard several common excuses why my clients are not taking the time to care for themselves—that is, to do self-care activities that are likely in their best interest. These excuses, which often masquerade as reasons, include the following:

- "I'm too busy."
- "I don't have time to _____." (Fill in the blank with a beneficial activity.)
- "I have to take care of the kids."
- "I have to take care of my spouse."
- "I have too many things to do around the house."
- "I have a lot of job responsibilities."
- "If I don't do it, then who will?"
- "I would feel guilty."
- "I've been so busy that I've never thought about self-care."
- "I have no idea what to do / what I would like to do for self-care."

I am not saying that these aren't legitimate responses for not creating time for self-care. As a matter of fact, not only is this typically the way clients feel, but it's often a pretty accurate picture of their situations. However, everything we do has consequences. Some of our actions yield positive results, while others, not so much. None of us are machines; we are human beings, which means although we're capable of accomplishing a lot, we all have limitations.

There are some who will read this and know in their heart that the pace at which they're currently going, and the number of things they're trying to juggle, is not sustainable. For many, it is unrealistic to continue trying to manage the number of tasks and the accompanying stress that comes from thinking they can do it all.

Too much stress can easily lead to anxiety, mood instability, increased tearfulness, insomnia, panic attacks, burnout, irritability, and depression, as well as physical symptoms such as chest pain, digestive issues (including ulcers), headaches, high blood pressure, body aches, a compromised immune system, and the aggravation of previous physical issues.

PRIORITIZING SELF-CARE

Engaging in self-care activities, or activities that you enjoy, does not require an elaborate plan. I've had clients who think that when I talk about self-care, I mean taking a trip to a tropical island or finding a new time-consuming or expensive hobby (which is fine and can be great, but only if it's practical for you). Sometimes taking care of oneself means doing simple, inexpensive things that can still yield huge benefits.

These simple self-care activities could include going for a walk, reading a good book, taking a bath, or sitting on a park bench watching the sun set. Often, it's just a matter of taking a pause from the hustle and bustle that surrounds us on a regular basis. It's giving ourselves a break, allowing our minds an opportunity to rest by focusing on something else besides our typical day-to-day stresses, and creating a sense of inner peace. In a few moments I will identify some specific interventions that may help with managing stress, achieving that sense of peace, and improving one's quality of life overall.

A part of caring for oneself is being aware of what we are putting into our minds and our bodies. Knowingly or unknowingly, we are constantly feeding ourselves things that are either beneficial or harmful (or at least *potentially* harmful). Most of us have heard plenty of messages encouraging us to avoid or reduce our intake of junk food (highly processed food that is high in sugar, salt, calories, and fat). It's widely known that these foods can cause significant health issues.

You've probably even heard this philosophy expressed in the saying "Garbage in, garbage out." I strongly believe this also applies to what we focus on and feed our minds. If a person is only watching excessive amounts of violent television shows, video games, and movies, and only listening to music that is angry or aggressive, it's hard to imagine that this will not compromise their ability to feel at peace with themselves and the world around them. True self-care involves taking good care of our body, mind, and spirit. When we are able to do this, it is easier to create an environment for growth and healing not just within ourselves but also within our society.

Taking the time to do things for yourself is a great way to demonstrate that you care about yourself. It shows that you are willing to do for yourself what you may have hoped someone else would have done for you. Be willing to make time for yourself, treat yourself, take yourself out for a good meal, or simply do those things that make you happy and bring you joy. Honor yourself and praise yourself for all that you've accomplished and overcome (recently or at any time in the past). I often encourage my clients to do these things for themselves as part of their overall treatment, in addition to working on their issues.

Self-care also includes speaking words of positivity to yourself. Feel free to tell yourself, "I like me." Better yet, say, "I love me." Even if someone doesn't truly believe these words at the time, I think if they're said often enough, there's a strong likelihood that a day will come when the words ring true. There is a point in my daily morning ritual where I always say, "I love me!" And I say it with conviction.

THE MIND-BODY-SPIRIT CONNECTION

Let me first say that there are many specific interventions or activities that fall under self-care. There is no one thing that works the same for everyone. When I'm in a session, I make suggestions or brainstorm with the client various things they may want to do and then try to help them choose what feels right and what may be the most beneficial.

With most of my adult clients, whether it's an individual or couple, I help them examine what they do (or don't do) to take care of their minds, bodies, and spirits. This is where I take a deep dive to discover if, when, and how they nurture these distinct components of their being. This is an important step in addressing whatever it is that led them to therapy. What does it really mean to "nurture" one's mind, body, and spirit? Let's take a look at this and how I approach each of these areas with my clients.

1. *Nurturing our minds*

Nurturing *our minds* means we are doing things that provide opportunities for our minds to be stimulated and to grow, such as engaging in hobbies, reading a book, going back to school, pursuing a new interest, or learning a new skill. The objective here is to do things that are unlike what usually occupies your thoughts. These tend to be things that add what I call "spice" to one's life, much in the same way we add seasoning to a meal we're cooking. We may not need to add the spices, but it sure does taste better when we do. Otherwise, we're left with a meal that's a little on the bland side.

Nurturing one's mind also means being aware of what we're putting into it. Are the things we're taking into our minds providing positive results, or are they producing toxicity? Are they assisting with personal growth, or are they just helping us escape the reality of our current situation? Are the things we're putting in our heads helping us to feel good or amplifying our pain?

Feeding our minds can yield a variety of benefits, including feeling more engaged and happier. Nurturing our minds can help us to feel a greater sense of balance, especially between what we feel we have to do and the many things we want to do. Taking care of our minds may even help us to be more prepared to deal with life's unexpected situations.

2. *Nurturing our bodies*

When it comes to nurturing *our bodies*, the benefits are fairly obvious. Again, keep in mind that everything is not for everybody. Having said that, when I explore this area with a client, I'm trying to discover what they do to take care of their actual physical body, producing positive or negative results. It is my hope they understand that if they don't take care of their body and their overall physical health, there is a greater chance they will eventually have to deal with unfortunate consequences. Nurturing our bodies includes, but is not limited to, making sure we are getting enough rest, eating a healthy and well-balanced diet, drinking plenty of water, and avoiding possible toxins, such as alcohol and cigarettes.

I also ask questions to determine if my clients are exercising on a consistent basis. If they admit they are not, then I inquire if are they getting *any* movement on a regular basis. Even if someone is not hitting the gym three to four times a week, some movement is better than no movement. Do they go for walks with their dog? Do they have a job that is physically demanding or includes opportunities for exercise?

You've probably heard the phrase "Use it or lose it." I believe this applies to our body's strength, flexibility, and internal systems. If we don't engage the many and various parts of our body, it's possible our health and overall abilities will decline. Movement is a sign of life and vitality. I strongly urge everyone, as much as they are able, to exercise or at least get

their body moving as often as possible. Also, if you are thinking about starting a committed exercise routine, speak to a
doctor first in case you have any underlying health issues that
need to be examined prior to beginning. This is what I advise
all my clients as well.

3. *Nurturing our spirit*

Last but not least is the value of nurturing *our spirit*. I often
ask my clients what, if anything, they are doing to feed their
spirit. They usually tell me about their level of involvement
as it relates to church or other religious activities. I then
explain that, although spirituality can be associated with a
church or religion, that is not what I meant by my question.
For me, taking care of one's spirit means engaging in activities that create or promote feelings of inner peace. Yes, going
to church and reading religious texts can produce feelings of
inner peace. However, I'm specifically referring to activities
that promote a sense of calm and ease, such as listening to
pleasant music, meditating, doing yoga, praying, or taking a
warm, relaxing bath.

I believe one of the best ways, and definitely one of my favorite ways, to nurture the spirit is to experience nature. There
are very few things that compare to going on a beautiful hike,
walking on a beach, sitting near a stream, visiting waterfalls,
or being out at night, staring up at a full moon or a sky filled
with twinkling stars. I haven't been able to experience it personally, but I've heard amazing things from people who've vis-
ited beautiful locations like the Grand Canyon, Yellowstone
National Park, or one of the numerous breathtaking mountain
ranges scattered around the world. I personally enjoy experiencing the beauty of a tropical island. (My wife and I love
Aruba.)

Traveling to one of these spectacular locations is not the

only way to enjoy nature. This could also be something as simple as sitting on a park bench watching tree branches swaying in the wind or watching a sunset or sunrise. I think it's unfortunate that every day there is a beautiful sunrise and sunset that most of us, including me, tend not to appreciate because we are too busy with our day-to-day lives. I also enjoy the smell in the air before the rain, as well as the flashes of lightning off in the distance at night.

I'm sure many would agree that there is something calming about being in nature. It's no wonder people often go to the beach and sit under an umbrella intending to read, only to fall fast asleep. It's no surprise that some of us enjoy waking up before sunrise in order to get to our favorite watering hole to fish. Sometimes just getting a cup of coffee or tea and staring out the window creates wonderful feelings of peace. I feel like the moments in which we unplug are necessary to help us be able to navigate the challenges we find ourselves having to deal with.

Taking the time to invest in ourselves and in our own wellness is extremely vital. Realistically, many of us may struggle to feed our mind, body, and spirit consistently or sufficiently. But I believe the more you strive to do so, the more likely you'll be successful.

Think of your mind, body, and spirit like three legs of a stool. If only two of the legs are sturdy, you might find it a little challenging to sit on it comfortably. Likewise, if you are only nurturing, say, your mind and your spirit but totally neglecting your body, you may find yourself out of balance without understanding why. In no way am I saying being balanced in all three areas is easy to do. However, I am suggesting that it's worth the effort to try. We all benefit from taking the time to try to nurture our mind, body, and spirit.

FINAL THOUGHTS ON SELF-CARE

There are a plethora of tools and activities that clients have shared that helped them take better care of themselves. Some have found activities such as gardening, painting, drawing, crafting, photography, restoring furniture, taking naps, or journaling to be very beneficial.

Whether you spend time in nature, express gratitude, or are simply aware of how your thoughts impact your emotional well-being, there are self-care dos and don'ts that can enhance your sense of inner peace. Below, I've provided a list of things you may want to do more of, followed by a list of things you may want to consider reducing or eliminating altogether.

Self-Care Dos

This is not an exhaustive list; however, some of the things here have already been suggested, and some are new. Hopefully they will help you or someone you know in navigating life's stressors:

- Spend quality time with friends and family.
- Establish boundaries (say no, if appropriate) when others are making demands of you that are compromising your mental, emotional, or physical health.
- Be patient with yourself.
- Forgive yourself.
- Reward or treat yourself for your hard work, accomplishments, or just hanging in there.
- Speak kind and loving words to yourself.
- Pray or meditate (if this matches your belief system).

- Laugh as often and as hard as you possibly can.
- Play more, whether it's with the dog, the children, the grandchildren, your partner, or by yourself!

Self-Care Don'ts

Now let's take a look at some things you may want to try to avoid or *not do*. Realistically, you may not be able to totally eliminate these items from your life, but I don't see anything wrong with trying to minimize the frequency at which you do them:

- Don't spend time (or at least reduce the time you spend) with those who drain or hurt you (mentally, emotionally, and physically).
- As much as realistically possible, avoid fighting, debating, or arguing with people (especially if it doesn't lead to a positive, healthy, or beneficial conclusion).
- Don't be so hard on yourself.
- Don't judge or criticize others (or at least don't allow yourself to do so to a point where you are angry or frustrated and your inner peace is compromised).
- Don't complain so much.
- Don't allow yourself to be overly concerned about how others may view you. (The late Johnnie Coleman, who was a minister of a church I used to attend, would always say, "What people think of me is none of my business.")

You may not agree with some of the items listed above.

However, these are simply my suggestions based on personal experience and what my clients have found to be beneficial.

Becoming Consistent

Several times throughout this book, I have stressed the value of being consistent. I don't believe I can overstate its importance, especially as it relates to accomplishing goals and achieving personal growth. I believe what we do often, we will get better at. Unfortunately, this is true whether we engage in positive thoughts and empowering patterns of behavior, or we frequently harbor toxic thoughts about ourselves, leading to poor decisions. We reinforce whatever it is that we decide to focus on in our lives.

There was a time in my life when I realized that meditation and yoga would be beneficial for me. So I would get up in the morning and try to spend at least twenty minutes doing each. There were plenty of times when I just didn't get it done—neither one. It was common for me to wake up later than I had planned and spend the rest of the morning quickly getting dressed, out the door, and off to work. It was during these instances when I would tell myself, "Well, maybe tomorrow." Often tomorrow became tomorrow, and the day after tomorrow. On average, I would meditate and do yoga anywhere from two to three times a week—too inconsistent to produce the feel-good results I was hoping for. I felt undisciplined, like I wasn't able to accomplish my goal of doing these things at least five days a week.

However, after attending a four-day motivational self-improvement retreat, I returned feeling renewed and determined. I told myself that I was going to meditate and do yoga not just five days a week but every day, seven days a week. Initially, it took a good deal of determination, discipline, and intentionality.

But after about two to three months, it became part of my daily routine, a habit no different from brushing my teeth or bathing. At this point in my life, it would feel very odd *not* to start my day doing these things. It's now part of my "hour of power." Into this hour, in addition to meditating and doing yoga, I've incorporated reading from at least two different books that are either spiritual, motivational, or autobiographical—pretty much anything that helps get me mentally and emotionally prepared for a new day. I believe that if we can demonstrate self-care on a consistent basis, we will become better equipped to deal with the problems that pop up in our lives.

As challenging as it may be, self-care is extremely important for those who take care of others. Some of us have jobs or responsibilities that are all about serving and helping others. As rewarding as this is, it can also be draining, both physically and mentally. Those of us in these positions compromise our ability to successfully do our jobs if we are not taking time out to rest and take care of our own emotional well-being. And for those of us who don't have careers in service but rather find ourselves responsible for family members—including kids, aging parents, or loved ones with disabilities—self-care is just as important.

I realize that for many of us, our days are filled with obligations, and our tendency is to prioritize taking care of others first. But the reality is, if we burn out or become incapacitated, not only are we negatively impacted, but those we serve may not get the assistance they need. Contrary to what some may believe, self-care does not mean being selfish. If you're a caregiver, please don't forget to give yourself some of the time, attention, care, and love that you give to others.

Don't Forget to Breathe

When it is difficult to find the time, the motivation, the

discipline, or the right interventions for self-care, there is one thing we can all do: breathe. When life's daily stressors become too difficult or overwhelming, breathing is something we all can do anytime and anywhere. Taking deep, long, and slow breaths can help us become centered and calm, allowing us to see our situation with increased clarity. Taking deep breaths can also help us identify solutions or help us to communicate more effectively. There are many scenarios in which people take deep breaths before they begin a task, whether it's a basketball player about to make an important free throw, or a speaker who is about to take the stage. Breathing can help with regaining composure, being more mindful, becoming still, and getting into a state of mind that makes situations more manageable and less stressful.

CHAPTER 8

Challenges in Treatment

From the beginning to the end, life is a school, complete with individualized tests and challenges.

—Elisabeth Kübler-Ross and David Kessler

During my twenty-plus years providing therapy to a variety of individuals and families, I have learned that some situations and people are more challenging than others. Every situation is unique, as is each person, which is why we require a variety of interventions and supports. This comes with the territory of being a mental health professional. However, that doesn't mean that clinicians don't find themselves in sessions where they tell themselves, "Guess I'll be earning my pay today."

These challenging situations have required me (and likely other mental health professionals) to be open-minded, creative, intuitive, knowledgeable, empathetic, and flexible in determining how to help or interact with clients. Some of these difficult scenarios include:

- those who have been victims of physical, emotional, or sexual abuse (especially if they're children or adolescents)
- those who are currently dealing with suicidal ideation
- those with a history of self-injurious behaviors (cutting, hair-pulling, self-abuse)
- those with addictions (drugs, alcohol, sex, pornography, gambling, overspending)
- those with severe or ongoing depression
- those with debilitating anxiety
- kids in foster care (especially those who have been there for a significant period of time)
- those who are struggling with the loss of a loved one

Of course, every individual is different, which means that the therapeutic intervention that may help one person may not help the next, despite them dealing with a similar issue. In this chapter I will share some of the things I've learned while working with individuals and families who unfortunately found themselves trying to navigate some of the above situations.

CHALLENGES TREATING THOSE DEALING WITH GRIEF AND LOSS

Whether personally or professionally, trying to be there for those who have lost a loved one is extremely difficult. I'm sure we've all seen or known people who were so distraught that they appear to be wrapped in a blanket of pain and grief. The death of someone who has played an important role in our lives can be very difficult to deal with and move on from.

Imagine you are a licensed professional counselor or therapist. A solemn single parent walks into your office. They sit down and sadly begin telling you their newborn child died recently. Perhaps they are struggling to maintain eye contact as they tear up, and their voice cracks while they share with you the events that took place and led to their overwhelming grief.

Even if you're not a mental health professional, and instead you're hearing this information from a family member, friend, or coworker, what do you say? What do you do? For most of us, whether we're licensed mental health professionals or not, it is difficult to come up with words that will comfort a person dealing with losing a loved one, especially losing a child. Typically, the first thing that comes to mind is something like, "I'm so sorry to hear about your loss." Or "Is there anything I can do for you?" Or "I'll be praying for you." These statements may sincerely come from the heart. However, we also know that despite our good intentions, they don't take away the pain of the person who is grieving. Many of us are simply not sure what to say at that moment. As a therapist, when someone is coming to me for help with their pain, I must try to find the right words to say or the right actions to take in order to support them and provide comfort.

Unfortunately, there are no magic phrases I have found that can instantly heal a person who is dealing with the loss of someone they deeply cared for. I've had to counsel not only those who have lost a child but also those who have lost their spouse, a parent, a close friend, a coworker, or even a beloved pet.

Working with Those Who Are Grieving

Although there are many stages of grief (denial, anger, bargaining, depression, acceptance), each person is likely to have their own way of mourning. It's important to accept each person's individual process, which includes the intensity of their pain and the time it takes for them to pass through any particular stage of grief.

If I have a client dealing with grief and loss, I typically do the following during our sessions:

- Be patient with the client and their grieving process.
- Encourage them to be patient with themselves.
- Listen with an empathetic ear.
- Take the time to learn about the person they lost and the relationship they shared.
- Explore with them what they may need in this moment, this session, this day, or this week (from me as their therapist and from others). Due to the pain they're experiencing, they may not yet know or be able to verbalize their needs.
- Encourage self-care by identifying ways they can take care of themselves at this time, whether it be emotionally, physically, or spiritually.
- Inquire about any religious beliefs they have. If they do subscribe to certain views, incorporate those into the session and their healing process.

As I mentioned previously, each individual and each situation is different. I have to be as open-minded as possible when trying to help and support a person dealing with grief and loss.

CHALLENGES TREATING THOSE
WHO HAVE BEEN ABUSED

A general definition of abuse is when a person is treated in

cruel and possibly violent ways. Abuse is likely to be significantly more damaging if it is done repeatedly or over an extended period of time. There are, of course, various types of
abuse, but the most common are physical, verbal, sexual, and
emotional. Child abuse is typically given its own category and
is particularly heartbreaking to encounter, not to mention it is
a serious crime.

I define physical abuse to be when a person is struck or hit
in an aggressive manner, typically causing pain. Sexual abuse
can be anything from inappropriately touching someone (especially one's genitals without their consent) to sexual assault
and rape.

Then there is the type of abuse that doesn't get the attention it deserves, which is emotional abuse. In this case a victim
could be dealing with a variety of toxic situations, including
being taken advantage of, told things that are hurtful, threatened, degraded, or gaslighted. With gaslighting, the perpetrator psychologically manipulates a person, causing them to
question their thoughts, their reality, and even their sanity.
This form of abuse causes significant mental and emotional
distress and can be tricky for the victim to identify at first.

Child abuse is usually defined as a child being mistreated
through physical and sexual abuse (which can take the form
of exploitation), child endangerment, emotional abuse, or
neglect. Anyone who causes a child to feel significant pain,
distress, and trauma is likely committing a crime. An adult
harming a child could lead to a variety of outcomes, including
a parent or guardian losing custody of their child, being fined,
or possibly even being imprisoned. A child being mistreated
and abused will not only be significantly and negatively impacted in the present, but also feel harmful effects well into
adulthood.

Adults can also be victims of abuse. I'm specifically speaking of elder abuse and the abuse inflicted upon those with

disabilities. Elder abuse typically occurs when someone intentionally causes harm to or takes advantage of an older adult (usually someone age sixty-five or older) or puts their overall well-being and safety at risk. Senior citizens, as well as those with disabilities, are vulnerable to being manipulated by people seeking to get ahold of their money or personal possessions. I've been made aware of instances where a family member was secretly siphoning money from their elderly parent's or grandparent's accounts. Some people even intercept the checks of the elderly and cash them for themselves. Then, of course, there is the endless number of scams that target vulnerable people who are susceptible to deception. This can occur while they're out in the community, when they answer the phone (where the person on the other end is either using encouragement or fear to get their money), or when they access the internet, through scams designed to get ahold of their finances. No matter how the scam is conducted, the damage can be quite significant and potentially devastating. In addition to losing their hard-earned money—something they desperately need in their final years—their mental and emotional health is also at risk of being compromised.

Neglect is another form of abuse that happens when a caregiver refuses or fails to provide basic needs, such as food, water, shelter, and medical care, to a point where it threatens the well-being of an elderly person or an individual with a disability.

In the United States, anyone can report the above-described forms of abuse. There's the National Child Abuse Hotline (1-800-422-4453) as well as local children and family service offices that are available to take calls when children are being abused. For the elderly and disabled, directly calling 911 or the police is another way of informing the authorities that a vulnerable person is being harmed.

When it comes to abuse, there are those who are required

by law to report suspected child abuse, child sexual abuse, or elder abuse. This means that if these individuals are informed, observe, or suspect that abuse has occurred, they must notify the appropriate authorities. Individuals mandated to make reports of abuse include doctors, hospital personnel, dentists, nurses, schoolteachers, school administrators, school counselors, child welfare agency personnel, law enforcement personnel, and mental health professionals, as well as clergy, athletic coaches, and people providing services at shelters, among others.

When someone decides to see a therapist as a result of being a victim of abuse, the therapist must be prepared to deal with some significant challenges. I believe in order to address issues of abuse, a clinician will likely need to display a variety of skills, insight, empathy, and compassion. In order to truly serve the client and help them in the best ways possible, the therapist may have to consider obtaining the services of other agencies as well.

Working with Those Who Have Been Abused

The first big challenge for me is listening to what is likely a very unfortunate (if not disturbing) situation while also seeing the pain it has caused another human being. The cruel treatment that some people inflict on others is startling, upsetting, and at times horrific. However, as a therapist, no matter what I hear someone describe, I have to remain professional by listening attentively, trying to understand their experience, identifying ways to support them, determining what to do next, and creating interventions that can provide opportunities for healing and growth. As I'm listening, I aim to avoid having them relive the experience and to prevent them from becoming overwhelmed with emotion. I may need information about what they've been through, but not at the cost of them being retraumatized.

There is no one action that will guarantee success when it comes to helping someone work through the traumas caused by abuse. Each situation is as different as each individual who is sharing their story. We all respond to trauma differently, past or present; therefore we all need slightly different forms of help. Finding the right thing to do or say at the right time becomes a major goal for me, and likely for other mental health professionals as well. I also realize that I must be patient with clients and patient with myself, understanding that it may take time to see progress and healing.

In some instances, I may suggest support groups (in fact, these may be more beneficial than individual therapy). There are also other clinicians who have more experience or specialize in certain areas (grief, abuse). In these cases, I may refer a client to another professional who I believe will be of greater assistance. The goal should always be doing what is in the best interest of the client.

Ultimately, if I'm able to provide even some degree of comfort and support to the client, I am doing my job. If someone expresses to me that they are benefiting from our sessions, then I am grateful to have made a difference. It is during these times that even small victories affirm I am doing what I have been called to do: fulfilling my purpose to serve others and do what I can to help people heal.

CHALLENGES TREATING THOSE STRUGGLING WITH ADDICTION

It seems we are all susceptible to becoming addicted to something. We are human, after all! We seek pleasure of all kinds and in many different ways. As a matter of fact, almost anything that feels good can become addictive. Some of the feel-good things that we enjoy doing may actually be addictive despite the good they do, including working out, taking daily naps, staying hydrated, praying, meditating, and countless other things that serve or nurture our mind, body, and spirit.

Then there are the addictive things that produce harmful effects or significantly impact our lives (and the lives of those around us) in negative ways. In this case, I'm referring to things like addiction to drugs, alcohol, sex, pornography, shopping, smoking, food (particularly unhealthy foods), gambling, video games, and plastic surgery, to name a few.

Unfortunately, once a person becomes addicted to something, other areas of their life can become toxic, impaired, or damaged. The obsession to engage in the activity can compromise one's work life, relationships, and physical, mental, and emotional health.

Addictions can result in a person doing any of the following:

- Being late for work (or not showing up at all) and ultimately losing their job
- Frequently arguing or getting into confrontations (verbal or physical) with family, partners, or coworkers
- Spending money maintaining their addiction instead of taking care of the basic needs of their family (food, clothing, rent/mortgage)
- Experiencing symptoms of withdrawal when not engaged in the activity, causing other emotional issues such as depression and anxiety (in addition to physical signs of withdrawal due to drug or alcohol addiction)
- Losing a significant amount of time and energy in an effort to receive that pleasurable feeling or dopamine hit

Whether it's any of the above-listed behaviors or others that are just as harmful, treating those with addictions can be challenging for both client and therapist.

Working with Those Struggling with Addiction

> *The greater the obstacle the more glory in overcoming it.*

> —Molière

I initially ask questions in order to assess whether the individual is even aware that they have an addiction. The majority of people who are addicted to something, when questioned, deny or attempt to minimize it. These people, when confronted, say things like "It's not an issue for me. I can stop doing *it* at any time." Or "I just do *it* because _____." (This is where they make up what is likely an excuse to justify their behavior.) Whenever any of us has a problem, to solve it we must begin by admitting there is something that needs to be solved. If a person refuses to admit they have a problem, then how can it be addressed? If, however, they acknowledge their struggle with addiction, I then try to determine if they are truly willing to put in the work to make a change, as well as learn the reasons why they want to do so. When we have a strong enough why, I believe almost anything is possible.

Once they've been open and honest enough to admit that they struggle with addiction, I seek to learn how it has negatively impacted their life and then proceed with exploring possible interventions to address their challenge.

If they are experiencing substance abuse issues, I will encourage them to seek out an addiction counselor and to consider going to a support group (such as Alcoholics Anonymous). A significant amount of evidence shows that group settings tend to be more beneficial than individual therapy for certain behaviors, including addictions. There are a variety of support groups out there, including twelve-step self-help groups, mutual support groups, and online groups.

There is something powerful and transformative that can happen when people come together with similar struggles. A person can then truly see that they are not alone. Also, a variety of ideas to move forward can come out of meetings. People will likely hear messages of hope and inspiration as others share how they have overcome, or continue to manage, their own addictions. As a therapist, whether a person chooses to go to a group session or not, I am strongly inclined to refer them out. This is where I will attempt to locate other clinicians in the community who are more qualified or better suited to help them, therefore increasing the likelihood they will overcome their addiction.

Therapists and counselors refer clients out for several reasons. Perhaps they have limited or no experience or training in treating individuals with certain diagnoses, the condition is outside of their scope of their practice, or they simply do not feel comfortable working with certain issues. It's also not uncommon for a client to see an addiction specialist while also working with a therapist like myself to address other issues, such as anxiety, depression, or relational challenges. Seeing two therapists is typically acceptable as long as they're working with the client in different and specified areas. This is the ethical thing to do in order to avoid what is called *duplication of services*: where two (or more) clinicians working with the same client are also working on the same issue. My bottom line as a therapist is simply to support the client with getting the help, the healing, and the tools they need to live a better life.

CHALLENGES TREATING THOSE WITH PHYSICAL HEALTH CONDITIONS

Treating a client who is experiencing significant amounts of pain or discomfort due to a physical health condition not only is challenging but also can be outright sad. Physical health conditions can cause a great deal of mental distress, including depression. I've worked with clients who had chronic back and joint pain, migraine headaches, and digestive issues and who have undergone surgeries (orthopedic, hysterectomies, etc.). But probably the most unfortunate are those who have had to fight one of the many forms of cancer.

When a Client Has Cancer

Although I wish this were not the case, I've had several clients (both adults and in one case a child) who were diagnosed with cancer, requiring them to undergo various procedures, including chemotherapy and radiation. Though I can try to help them mentally and emotionally, I feel limited regarding how much I can do to help their body physically fight cancer. I try to do all I can to provide a place for them to share their thoughts, emotions, feelings, and fears. It's not uncommon for clients to ask why this happened to them, as they try to wrap their head around this unfortunate condition.

I know I'm not the first person to ask this question, but why does it appear so often that bad things happen to good people? Why does the innocent child sitting before me have to endure leukemia or some other unfortunate health condition? I have no answers, but I will do everything in my power to help each person through the turbulent periods of their life.

A person may develop a variety of emotional challenges,

such as anxiety and depression, after they find out that they have cancer and must undergo the recommended treatments. Their self-esteem may also be negatively impacted, depending on how the treatments impact their body (hair loss, weight gain, weight loss, rashes, skin discoloration). It is my goal to assist them with managing those feelings as well as a host of others that may arise. Depending on the individual, I may try to be encouraging or to utilize resources such as articles, books, or videos to provide some hope, if not inspiration.

A lot of information seems to indicate that when one is battling cancer, a positive mental attitude is far more beneficial than a negative one. However, as with any other client, I have to determine along with the client what is best for them, which is often based on what they want or need the most.

CHALLENGES TREATING THOSE FEELING STUCK

Let me first define what I mean by someone feeling "stuck." These individuals may believe they are in a challenging situation, but they also feel helpless to change it. It's not uncommon for those with this mindset to feel there's absolutely nothing they can do about their circumstances. For some, this might mean not knowing what to do, not having the energy to take action, or feeling hopeless when it comes to making a change. They may feel stuck in a toxic relationship or in a job that may be sucking the very life out of them.

Then there are those who are stuck because they're afraid: afraid of what might or might not happen; afraid of the judgment of others; or afraid of the emotions, thoughts, and feelings that may arise and need to be dealt with.

Working with Someone Who Feels Stuck

Individuals who are stuck present challenges requiring unique goals and interventions. A person who is feeling this way may first need to adopt a mindset where they believe that hope is not lost; they *can* do something to change their circumstances. This is, of course, much easier said than done. But I find it helpful for people to be reminded about past situations that they endured and overcame.

We've all had challenges that may have felt insurmountable, but somehow we got through them. We may have moved on and forgotten all that we went through to come out on top. But these successes can serve as reminders of the strength and resiliency that we were able to demonstrate. That same ability to overcome is still there somewhere within.

I'm a firm believer that we are all co-creators of our individual worlds and lives, based on the thoughts we frequently have and the actions we frequently take. So in this case, one of my initial objectives is to help them believe in themselves (perhaps once again), believe in what is possible, and believe that they can do *something*. I want them to believe they can take a step toward creating positive change, no matter how insignificant it may appear. I typically try to help the client identify a small goal to create momentum and a belief that they are not powerless.

It's not uncommon for individuals who are feeling stuck to be overly critical toward themselves and negative about their situation. In this case, I'll make attempts to normalize their thoughts or challenge them by relating the experiences of others or even my own. I want them to realize that they're not alone, nor are they the only ones who have had to deal with their situation. And finally, I encourage them to be patient with themselves as well as with change. There are times when a person can change rapidly, if not in an instant, but I believe there are those who require more time.

Working with Someone Stuck in a Toxic Intimate Relationship

Someone who is *stuck* in a toxic or harmful relationship can be emotionally, mentally, and even physically drained. People in this situation often experience a lot of frustration directed at the other person or at themselves. It's not uncommon for this to open the door to anxiety or depression.

I feel it's important to discuss this feeling of being stuck in a negative or toxic relationship because of how often I have clients in this situation. My caseload almost always contains several people (often female) who are experiencing difficulty with ending a relationship that they know is causing them emotional misery and, in rare cases, resulting in them being a victim of physical violence. Typically, the stuck person has put up with numerous behaviors from their partner, including being disrespected, yelled at, cursed at, talked down to, lied to, cheated on, or unappreciated. Regardless of the mistreatment, they stay in the relationship, even if friends and family have tried desperately to get them to leave. At some point during the relationship, they've likely asked themselves, "Why am I staying in this?" or "Why do I continue putting up with this behavior?"

During my years as a therapist, I've worked with female clients who have gotten involved with married men. These women tend to acknowledge or logically know that they should not be in this relationship for several obvious reasons, including the fact that the man has violated the vows of his own marriage. It is very easy for an outsider to judge a woman for being in this situation. However, for the people to whom I've provided counsel, it's often far more complicated, and therefore they can't simply walk away. I do what I can to support where they are and try to find ways to help them create the inner strength to end the relationship and find someone who is worthy of their time, attention, and love.

From my experiences, I've learned that there are a variety of reasons why someone may remain stuck in an obviously unhealthy relationship:

- *Fear.* This includes the fear of being alone, the fear of what one person may do to the other or to their family if they try to leave, and the fear of what the other individual may do to themselves. (Sometimes the partner makes threats to hurt or kill themselves if the other decides to leave.) This also includes the fear of how leaving may negatively impact the kids (if there are children involved) and the fear of how they will be perceived by friends, family, or coworkers.
- *Codependency.* An individual may become codependent when they have become so accustomed to a partner being a part of their lives that they have unknowingly become addicted to that person's role or presence in their life. Perhaps they've always been in a relationship and are uncomfortable with the thought of being single or alone.
- *A focus on the positive attributes of the toxic person.* Despite knowing and having a clear understanding of the person's flaws, shortcomings, or issues, some remain in the relationship by focusing on the positive traits of the individual who is mistreating them.
- *A focus on the good times while minimizing the toxic or upsetting experiences.* Many ignore or play down the effects of extremely volatile or dysfunctional behaviors.

- *Denial.* I've seen people who were stuck in toxic relationships because it was easier to live in a state of denial than to accept the reality of their situation. They may refuse to believe that, despite how negative, toxic, and abusive the relationship is, this person is their soulmate. These people tend to be very reluctant to consider the possibility that they might be better off without this person. They may struggle with the idea that there are other people who are a much better match for them.
- *Financial dependency.* Some people remain stuck in a dysfunctional relationship because of money, especially if they are married or live together. These people may think that they will *not* be able to pay their bills if the other leaves. Perhaps the other person is the primary earner, there are children involved, or they simply don't know if they can meet their financial needs on their own if they were to leave.
- *A lack of ego strength.* Ego strength can be defined as having enough confidence or resiliency to deal with difficult or challenging situations. Some stay because they have not yet gained the strength to end the unhealthy relationship. I always have hope that in time, my clients eventually will, and I intend to do as much as I can to support them until then.
- *False hopes.* False hopes are beliefs that the relationship will get better despite the person never seeing signs of improvement or their partner never making efforts to improve.

Other unfortunate reasons include not loving themselves

enough and not having an example of what it means to be in a healthy relationship. No matter the reason, it can be very challenging for the client to get out of the dysfunctional situation and for the clinician to help them get to a place where they can heal and grow through it.

Working with Those Stuck in Damaging Relationships

Despite the challenge presented by a client who appears stuck, I believe I can help. First, I want to understand how they view their situation as well as the degree of hopelessness they may be experiencing. I want to learn the possible reasons why they're in the situation. During this time, I'm also searching for underlying causes, such as their past experiences or past traumas. Once this information is obtained, it's time for us to work collaboratively and seek all possible interventions that may help them to become unstuck. Hopefully, we can build momentum for them to move forward with the life they desire and deserve. As I've stated before, there is no one way to address every challenge. Each situation and each person should be taken into consideration as the therapist and client work to find solutions.

Those Stuck in a Toxic Work Environment

You probably won't be too surprised to hear this, but there are plenty of times where I see clients who feel they have limited options or are stuck in a bad job situation. It's common knowledge that, at least in America, work-related stress has deeply affected us emotionally, sometimes leading to burnout, physical ailments, or more severe issues like headaches, ulcers, or increased risk of heart disease. According to a survey from Everest College, 83 percent of US workers suffer from work-related stress.[1]

The anxiety and strain that we deal with in the workplace are often the result of demands and deadlines, as well as bosses who lack the skills to be both competent and compassionate leaders. In today's world, it seems employers demand more and more of their employees. People feel disrespected, undervalued, and treated like tools or pawns, only there to benefit the organization and maximize profits. Employers often expect their staff to work longer hours, or however many hours it takes to meet the company's goals.

In addition to the demands placed on staff by their superiors, other aspects of the work environment can contribute to its toxicity. Employees may find it difficult to do their jobs due to:

- mistreatment or disrespect from coworkers
- discrimination because of their age, sex, race, religion, sexual preference or identity, disability, or pregnancy
- bullying (management to subordinates)
- teasing/taunting (between management and staff or between coworkers)
- sexual harassment
- gossip
- unmotivated coworkers
- poor communication between employees and management
- lack of fair pay (based on the going rate for the position)
- anxiety due to fears of being terminated

Helping Those in Toxic Work Environments

One of the primary challenges when counseling individuals in these situations is that despite the harmful work environment, they may feel stuck and therefore can't leave. People remain in highly stressful job situations for many reasons. They likely need their job in order to pay their bills and take care of their family. Others may be worried about how long it will take to find another job if they quit their current one. Still others are concerned about whether a new job could pay enough, which is especially problematic if they are receiving a large salary in their current position. They may question themselves: "Will things get better somewhere else?" "What will my friends and family say?" "Will I look weak or like a quitter?" "How will this look on my resume?" "Is it even possible for me to find something better than this?"

As their therapist, I try to avoid telling a client what they should do. I would never say that they should quit, nor would I tell them they should stay. But what I will do is help them gain a clearer understanding of the situation and provide a place to process their feelings, explore options, and find ways to support whatever their decision is. If they decide to remain, I'll do my best to help them develop coping strategies to manage their workplace challenges. However, if they determine it is in their best interest to leave, then my goal will shift to assisting them with going forward confidently and identifying a possible plan of action.

CHALLENGES IN TREATING PEOPLE WITH SEVERE DEPRESSION

In chapter 2, I spent time discussing depression, its challenges, and its impact on people. For some dealing with depression, the struggle to manage their feelings is greater because of how debilitating and devastating it has been to their lives. Despite how difficult severe depression can be for these individuals, it can also be challenging for the clinician. The therapist has to consider how the client's lifestyle may be playing a role, as well as possible chemical imbalances in their brain. There are many researchers and clinicians who believe low levels of serotonin contribute to or cause depression. Depression and other health issues can also be inherited from family members. Therefore treating these individuals may require unique interventions, a greater understanding of depression's causes, and possibly more time to see progress.

As stated earlier in this book, I strongly recommend that an individual experiencing significant struggles with depression (or other diagnoses interfering with one's daily life) speak with their primary care physician or a psychiatrist in order to examine what is going on. A qualified doctor should be able to not only consider different options for medications but also explain how these medications work and address any questions the patient may have.

OTHER POSSIBLE CHALLENGES IN TREATMENT

A few other situations have been challenging and therefore required me to utilize a variety of therapeutic skills and professional experiences to help an individual, couple, or family:

Children in Foster Care

This is often an unfortunate, if not sad, situation. Every child who is "in the system" is there for a variety of reasons: Both the child and the family are in crisis. Perhaps they no longer or temporarily do not have family to care for them. Maybe they were taken away from the family due to physical abuse, sexual abuse, or neglect. I have had children as clients who were in foster care because their primary caretaker had addiction or substance abuse issues, preventing them from being a safe and effective parent. No matter the reason a child is in foster care, if they are my client, it becomes my job to support them therapeutically. Unfortunately, I have had clients in the system who moved from home to home, from one temporary family to another. Meanwhile, I was able to remain their clinician (usually by providing in-home therapy), being one constant aspect, if not the only one, of their young life. A foster child packing up their belongings in large black plastic bags as they prepare once again to be moved into a new placement is definitely not an easy thing to witness.

Teens Who Don't Want to Be There

Let's face it: teenagers can be challenging in or out of therapy. It's not uncommon for a parent to become aware of their adolescent's need to receive some type of treatment, but their child is not interested or perhaps doesn't even believe they need it. If the parent can get them to the first couple of sessions, I am usually able to get the adolescent to a point where they feel comfortable and safe and finally become a willing participant. However, there have been a few occasions when despite some progress in developing the therapeutic relationship, they stopped coming and the goals never materialized. Hopefully, they didn't give up on the idea of therapy and found greater success with another clinician.

A Couple Ending Their Marriage

I've had to learn to accept when a couple's issues are insurmountable. Despite the efforts made to save the relationship, they have decided to divorce and go their separate ways.

Seeing two people who loved each other at one point end their relationship is like a sad ending to a movie. However, I also acknowledge that splitting up is a reality for many couples.

Virtual Therapy Sessions

Due in large part to the COVID-19 pandemic, virtual therapy sessions have become commonplace in mental health care and treatment. For the majority of the clinicians I know, anywhere from 60 to 100 percent of their sessions are now done via a video screen or perhaps the telephone. Many clients appear to like the convenience of virtual sessions. They get to remain in the comfort of their own home (or their car or office) and avoid the commute they must endure when going to a physical office.

The challenge is not that the quality of the therapeutic service is being compromised, but more so about the technology and where the client is when the session is taking place. With so many therapy sessions occurring virtually, it has become obvious that everyone uses different devices, some of which are older than others. Some clients live in homes or areas that have poor Wi-Fi service, have an old router, or are too far away from the router to maintain a clear signal. It can definitely become frustrating when I'm desperately trying to hear what the client is saying as their image or voice becomes choppy or distorted.

While conducting therapy sessions virtually, I have also been interrupted by phone calls, family members, pets, or outside noises (e.g., sirens and lawn equipment). And finally, many activities or therapeutic interventions that I've used in the past have had to be revised or eliminated because they are only appropriate for face-to-face, in-person sessions.

Regardless of the situation or the person, I accept and remain open to the challenges that may present themselves when trying to conduct therapy sessions. Every career has areas where things can get difficult from time to time, and this is also true for therapists. There are, of course, other situations that can be difficult for counselors. Please know that just because I've identified a few here doesn't mean they're insurmountable or that I don't welcome both the challenge and the opportunity to help improve someone's life. As long as the client is willing to put in the necessary effort and work with me to overcome their issues, I believe positive change can occur.

CHAPTER 9

Concerns for Our Communities and World

We must learn to live together as brothers or perish together as fools.

—Martin Luther King Jr.

I thoroughly enjoy teaching my introduction to psychology class every semester at a community college in Georgia. It meets twice a week for an hour and twenty minutes. I do my best to provide opportunities for my students to learn not only about the world of psychology but also more about people and themselves. Along the way, I also hope they improve their critical-thinking skills and gain new perspectives on how to deal with life and the challenges that will come their way. I often show motivational videos for the first few minutes of class as an additional way to inspire them to overcome their personal trials and achieve their goals. Throughout the semester, the students are encouraged to share their thoughts; be attentive, respectful listeners to their classmates; and be open to considering the opinions of others.

I have had the pleasure of teaching some wonderful students; however, as we get deeper into each semester and our connection grows, there are times when I'm concerned about their future. I try to be as open-minded as possible when they disclose their thoughts, experiences, and beliefs. They often share wonderful opinions and amazing stories, but I also hear how many of them are struggling with various aspects of their life.

Some of the challenges that students have shared include difficulties with their jobs, school, relationships, money, and families. I worry when they talk about being overwhelmed or having difficulties managing anxiety or depression. I get concerned when it appears many of them are struggling to either develop intimate, loving relationships or remain in them. Based on what I hear in the classroom (as well as in my sessions), I often wonder, *What is truly important to them? What is the foundation of their morals and values?*

Unfortunately, my concerns for future generations go beyond the students in my classroom; I have quite a few other concerns as well. It's likely some of my concerns are similar to your own, whether you're a mental health professional or not—legitimate worries about your personal life, the lives of your loved ones, your career, your health, your finances, and the overall state of the world.

This chapter will primarily focus on some of the patterns, behaviors, and events I see in our society that have led me to believe that there are some things we could and should be doing better, or at the very least *differently*. Some I've presented in the form of questions, while others are my personal thoughts and observations. I'm not identifying these things to scare anyone; instead, I hope they serve as a wake-up call for some of the issues that we need to address sooner rather than later. If we can agree to work on these areas together as a society, I believe we can find solutions that produce positive change for individuals, families, and communities.

We all need to accept certain realities. I feel we should recognize our issues without catastrophizing them or believing they are the downfall of society. Instead, perhaps we should view some of our struggles as opportunities to rise, grow, and create a world that aligns with our truest and greatest potential. I committed myself to living a life of service to others; otherwise, I would never have decided to devote my life to working as a therapist. When it comes to positive change, anything is possible, but we must be willing to think and act differently; otherwise, things will remain as they are or perhaps get even worse.

IS SOCIETY DOING ENOUGH TO HELP THOSE STRUGGLING WITH MENTAL ILLNESS?

Many people, myself included, are concerned about the hypocrisy of politicians, government leaders, and the medical community who talk about the importance of mental health services and yet fail to consistently implement them for everyone, not just those with the financial means to obtain treatment. Despite our nation's mental health crisis frequently being in the media spotlight, increasingly high numbers of people still struggle with depression, anxiety, addiction, anger, and suicidal thoughts.[1] Is society truly doing what is necessary to ensure people are getting the treatment many so desperately need? I believe the answer is a resounding no. And here's why.

Accessibility

According to the National Alliance on Mental Illness, nearly half of the sixty million adults and children with mental health issues in the United States go without treatment.[2] The reasons vary, but often it is the result of inaccessibility, including limited locations to receive therapy and a lack of affordable health care or the financial means to pay out of pocket.

I have witnessed many occasions when a client with health insurance is met with their own barriers to receiving therapy. Some insurance companies limit the number of therapy sessions a person can have within a given timeframe. If treatment goes beyond a certain timeline, some insurance companies start questioning the necessity of continuing the service. I have had clients—despite me completing the necessary paperwork for ongoing care and speaking with insurance representatives over the phone—whose insurance companies state they will no longer be paying for sessions. In these situations, they didn't explain to me (at least not in a way that makes sense) why they made their decision, which leads me to believe their rationale is about their bottom line; they simply no longer want to spend additional money treating this client.

Some insurance companies have become difficult for mental health professionals to work with due to low reimbursement rates or the arduous, time-consuming paperwork they want completed. As a result, many clinicians have increasingly decided not to take insurance of any kind. This becomes a headache for those seeking therapy when they contact a therapist only to discover that not only is their insurance not accepted, but payment must be made with cash or a credit card in full on the day of service. We are now seeing similar challenges with doctors and dentists, who often make changes regarding the insurance they accept, forcing patients to go "out of network" and pay for the service themselves.

What about the approximately thirty million Americans who have no health insurance? Yes, there are services out there that may provide therapy pro bono or calculate fees on a sliding scale (a discounted fee based on the client's ability to pay). For some, Medicaid is also a possibility.

One affordable option is a facility where interns/trainees conduct therapy under the supervision of a licensed professional. These sessions may be free or offered at a significantly reduced fee because they are provided by individuals who typically don't have as much experience or who have yet to become fully licensed. Despite the counselor's experience in providing therapy, they can be just as beneficial and helpful as someone who has been doing it for a longer period of time.

Despite the attempts of some to make mental health accessible, I don't believe enough is being done. As a society, we need to find ways to provide everyone with mental health services, especially in a time of need, regardless of their ability to pay. Fortunately, we have crisis hotlines and other resources in various communities to help people, but I believe we can do a lot more, and we should.

The Unmet Mental Health Needs of Students

Some schools employ a nurse (at least part-time) to address the physical issues that may pop up for students during the day and throughout the year. Most schools also have school counselors and at least one school psychologist. However, this is nowhere near the amount of mental health support today's elementary, junior high, and high school students need.

According to an article in the *Archives of General Psychiatry*, "One in five children and youth have a diagnosable emotional, behavioral or mental health disorder, and one in ten young people have a mental health challenge that is severe enough to impair how they function at home, school or in the community."[3] Given these numbers, it's vitally important that we figure out how to help our kids more than we currently are. Our society has made it difficult for children to manage their thoughts, their worlds, and their environments. They are often overwhelmed, lack coping skills, and are negatively impacted by situations that are out of their control. We also have to consider the things that they're consumed by, such as social media, materialism, and violence in films and TV, and the negative consequences that these produce.

I believe that every elementary, middle, and high school should employ full-time mental health employees. They would, of course, help when a student is in crisis, but their primary focus would be to provide weekly individual and group therapy sessions to those most at risk. Parents would have to sign consent forms to treat, but they would know that their child's mental and emotional issues are being addressed on a regular basis. This would be very beneficial, if not convenient, for parents whose work schedules make it difficult for them to take their children to see a therapist. This would also help families who either don't have insurance or lack the ability to pay for therapy sessions.

You may feel that schools already have psychologists who do this, but as with most things, it's not that simple—and in many cases, it's not possible. School psychologists can do assessments, testing, and evaluations, and work with administrators and teachers, all in an effort to create the best learning environment possible for students. They may also identify behavioral issues and learning difficulties affecting a student's ability to succeed academically. Despite all that they do, these responsibilities, combined with the number of enrolled students, make it virtually impossible for them to meet the emotional and mental health needs of an entire school.

Then there are the school counselors who are there to help the students be successful in school. Whether it's dealing with social or emotional needs, providing crisis counseling, having meetings or consulting with parents, addressing difficulties in the classroom, or referring them to services outside the school, the school counselor is there to help. However, because of the administrative duties that they are also responsible for, in combination with their extremely large caseloads, school counselors are not able to provide the level of care or mental health services that an entire school may need (which is why they may suggest that a parent take their child to receive outside therapy).

Success for All Students

I was fortunate to experience firsthand the positive effects of having licensed mental health professionals in schools. About ten years ago I was part of a school-based therapeutic program just outside of Atlanta. It was a federally funded five-year program called Success for All Students. Our staff consisted of about twenty-five licensed therapists, counselors, social workers, and interns; a substance abuse counselor; and a deputy sheriff; plus case managers and full-time administrative staff. From what I can recall, we were a team of about sixty to seventy people with one primary goal: to help children and teens by addressing their emotional and mental issues and other challenges that negatively impact their lives and their ability to achieve academic success.

I typically had anywhere from two to three public schools (depending on the specific school year) where I was responsible for helping students weekly by providing individual therapy sessions during their school day. These were students whom the school counselors or teachers identified as needing help and whose parents had already met with me to sign consent paperwork.

Every therapist in the Success for All Students program

was assigned to at least one high school. For me, this was where my home office was located. This was also where I got to experience firsthand the benefit of being a therapist located on a school's campus. You see, many of the counselors were overwhelmed with their responsibilities (as well as their extremely large caseloads), which made it very difficult to address an individual student's emotional challenges. If the counselors came across a student in need of mental health services who was also struggling academically, they would reach out to the parent and see if they were interested in having their child be a part of the program. Once a student entered the system, I would identify the right time to meet with them during their school day and begin keeping track of their grades.

We found that the majority of our school-based clients benefited, as evidenced by more emotional stability and improved grades. Because I was in the high school, students could take care of their emotional needs by obtaining a pass from their teacher and voluntarily coming to see me. If I was unavailable, they could leave a note in the hanging folder outside my office and I would get back to them as soon as I could.

I believe they appreciated and benefited from this convenience. Our therapeutic relationship made them feel so safe and comfortable that some of them told their friends about being in therapy with me. On a few occasions, in their free time (lunch, before holiday breaks when they were not doing lessons), they would come to chat, bring their peers, play UNO, or just hang out.

It's unfortunate that the program only lasted for five years and that it was only offered in a select area. During those years, our agency heard from many principals, teachers, school counselors, parents, and administrative staff how glad they were that we were there for the kids. As the program came to a close, many school officials expressed their disappointment that they would no longer be able to use our services.

The Success for All Students program proved what's possible and how impactful in-school therapy could be. Children need more support than ever before. If we implemented these programs in every school system at every grade level, grades would improve, behavioral problems would decrease, fewer young people would express thoughts of suicide, and school shootings committed by students could be eliminated.

Positive Signs for Therapy and Schools

There is some good news, however, because increasingly there are more schools working with clinicians in their community or hiring therapists to play a role within their institutions. There has also been an increase in federal policy measures (the Bipartisan Safer Communities Act and the American Rescue Plan Act of 2021) designed to provide pathways to support school-based mental health services with the goal of expanding and increasing access to mental health care in schools.

Most colleges and universities, regardless of size, also have mental health services that are available for free to both full-time and part-time students. This is a good thing; however, in my experience, most college students are unaware of these services or choose not to utilize them.

THE CURRENT STATE OF OUR SOCIETY

Another concern that has produced a lot of stress, anxiety, and likely a host of other mental health issues is our increasingly contentious behavior, which is often highlighted and even exaggerated on the news and on social media. Our society has become more combative, judgmental, and opinionated. We continue to divide ourselves into our own little groups, displaying what I consider a gang mentality or an "us against them" mindset.

Civility and respect for one another have taken a back seat, especially once we're angry or upset (which seems to happen pretty easily these days). Many of us have become extremely sensitive to opinions different from ours. Apparently, everyone seems to feel their opinion is fact. Perhaps it's just me, but I struggle to see many examples (in real life, on social media, on television, or in films) of forgiveness, compassion, or a willingness to understand one another—despite Alexander Pope's adage, "To err is human, to forgive divine."[4] We know logically that none of us are perfect, yet we minimize the fact that people should be given the opportunity to learn from their mistakes or questionable decisions. Why are we so much quicker to blame, judge, and criticize than we are to understand, uplift, and express love?

I find it ironic that many of the most divisive people are those who profess to worship or believe in a higher power. One whose existence I was always taught to believe personified forgiveness and love.

Our tendency to judge one another causes us to spend too much time venting about what we don't like (about a thing, a person, an idea, a belief, an event, or a group of people) and not enough time trying to work together to find solutions to our common problems. Our ignorance of the truth that we are all connected is a primary reason why we suffer as much as we do.

During sessions with clients who are struggling with anxiety or depression, there have been instances when they indicated feeling overwhelmed by what they see taking place in the world. We are all exposed to a barrage of information from the many networks, streaming channels, social media platforms, and national and local news outlets. If a person wants to, they can easily turn to one of several cable news channels and watch the same story twenty-four hours a day. Of course, there's nothing wrong with being informed about what's going on in our world; however, a vast majority of the information we are being fed is negative, dramatized, or designed to invoke fear or unease.

It's not hard to imagine why we struggle with anxiety, because our world seems to be spiraling out of control. The media always seems to make sure we know about every dramatic or traumatic situation taking place.

We are experiencing a lot of challenges in our society and our world. New issues seem to arise before we can resolve old ones. (I often wonder how much we're even trying to resolve them.) If not a mass shooting, there are one-on-one shootings every day. The rich are wealthier than ever while the poor get poorer (a.k.a. income inequality). We always seem to have more diseases to worry about, such as COVID-19, monkeypox, or something waiting on the horizon. Our politicians continue to create a greater divide between different parties and just can't seem to work together in the best interest of their citizens. There are also ongoing issues with racism, ageism, discrimination, and prejudice against people due to their gender/gender preferences or religion. Global climate change continues to produce extreme weather. We also continue to deal with our questionable, outdated education system; health care issues; rising childcare costs; corporate greed; selfishness; materialism; the safety of our food and water; and the ever-increasing need to address the mental health issues of people today.

This, of course, isn't everything society is trying to manage, but when we are forced to face such a litany of issues at the same time, one can see how easy it is to become overwhelmed.

The Divided States of America

Another concern that I hope everyone acknowledges is the

divisiveness of this nation. When people are living in fear, they tend to become distrustful of others. This then opens the door to people becoming less willing to help one another. They may become more selfish and focus solely on what they need, and not on others in the community (as was demonstrated by hoarding during the initial phases of the pandemic). This fear then produces a divided community, and I believe a divided community is a stressed-out and weakened one. We stop serving others and instead focus on serving ourselves. Whether we want to accept it or not, we are all connected. At some point and in some way, what affects one person can easily affect others. If we can overcome our differences and develop healthy and trusting relationships with our neighbors, we'll be stronger together than we could ever be apart.

Perhaps our tendency to separate ourselves from one another is due in part to a desire to feel elevated above others. So many of us seem to believe we are in some way better than another person or group of people. Unfortunately, many who believe that they are special see others as less-than and therefore find ways to diminish them.

Living in mistrust and division only solidifies suffering within our society. Our lack of trust is simply a manifestation of our fears, which causes us to experience both internal and external unrest.

Being Busy, Stressed, and Disconnected

For many in the US, our lives have become busier than ever. Growing up, I was told that advances in technology would make things easier. We'll have more free time for the things that really matter, like being with friends and relaxing. However, that does not appear to be what is happening. Instead, it is not uncommon for a person to take a full-time job where they are expected to work forty hours a week, only to find they must work much more. A lot of people are working longer days and doing job-related tasks over the weekend. Some find themselves taking work with them on their vacation. These efforts are typically not rewarded financially. Whether there is monetary gain or not, working additional hours and sacrificing our free time comes at the cost of burnout and compromised mental and physical health.

Becoming consumed with our careers can easily lead to a reduction in quality time and meaningful interactions with others. I've had clients who have struggled to navigate work and family demands, causing them to completely eliminate spending time with their friends or having a social life.

By nature we are social creatures, and to varying degrees we benefit from interacting with others. When I go too long without connecting with people, my mood and energy level tend to go down. Sometimes I'm not fully aware of what's happening, or why I'm feeling out of sorts and sad. Ultimately, through self-examination and maybe after having conversations with my wife, I gain a greater awareness of what's taking place: I've gone too long without connecting with others. It's not long after that I make it my business to reach out and reconnect with friends or a family member whom I haven't spoken to in a while.

Some people, in an effort to address loneliness and isolation, are compelled to pursue artificial relationships, or a sense of closeness that comes through social media or even video games. Now I'm not saying that these are not beneficial and can't produce positive effects. However, this may not be enough for some of us to feel truly connected to others.

Final Concerns

In addition to the issues I've already cited, there are quite a few other things I worry about as a therapist and as a human being. Perhaps some of the following concern you as well:

- Both the short- and long-term effects of so many children and young people being exposed to pornography (which is consumed at epidemic proportions yet is rarely discussed).
- The increasing value we place on money, materialism, and acquiring *stuff*. As a result, we seek happiness outside of ourselves instead of taking the time to look within and find what we are truly most in need of.
- People's (especially the younger generation's) seeming reluctance to accept responsibility for their actions; instead they place the blame on others.
- Unknown and underreported physical abuse, sexual abuse, neglect, and sex trafficking against children in this country and the world.
- The ever-increasing frequency in which people use drugs and alcohol to cope with life stressors, including those that are both risky and dangerous, like cocaine and fentanyl, not to mention those who feel the need to use drugs to have a good time while hanging with friends.
- The never-ending gun violence in America, which is too often the result of people choosing to resolve a temporary problem with a permanent solution. People use guns to retaliate or feel empowered. Some are so paranoid and fearful that they believe their only option is to shoot another human being, possibly ending a life.

- The increase in the number of individuals and families who cannot meet their basic needs, including shelter, access to medical care (including dental and mental health), healthy food options (or food in general), and clean drinking water.
- The path we're on destroying our communities and our planet. We harm our planet by polluting and destroying nature (the land, air, sea, and forests), making it unsafe or unable to sustain life. It usually takes humans far less time to destroy than it does to repair almost anything, so it's important that we gain a better understanding of the consequences of our actions in order to determine if we are hurting or healing, building or destroying our communities and the earth.
- Our outdated education system and teaching methods. This system, which has been around for over a hundred years, doesn't take into account the individual needs of children and the different ways in which they may learn. We don't appear to prepare students for the real world by teaching the skills they'll need when they're adults. We emphasize the wrong things in the classroom, and thus children spend little to no time learning to build wealth and be resilient, developing strong communication skills, developing creativity, learning trades (as they once did many years ago), and improving their critical-thinking or problem-solving skills. Instead, the school system's priority remains focused on standardized test scores, lectures, and note-taking for retaining information just long enough to take exams,

instead of truly understanding and learning the material.

- Our correctional system and its inability to rehabilitate people or to deter crime. I can't help but wonder if sending people to prison was ever meant to help those who made poor decisions. Of course, I'm not necessarily talking about those who've committed violent crimes but about those who have committed lesser offenses, who may go off to jail and thus become mentally or emotionally damaged only to come out of the system with more issues than when they went in. In today's world, it feels as if prison is simply a way of punishing people by taking them out of society, with no real intention to rehabilitate or prepare them for when their time has been served.

Although these are just some of the things that concern me based on my lifelong observations as a licensed marriage and family therapist, I do not want to come off sounding like a pessimist. That is not my intention. I believe that collectively we will make greater efforts to do the things in our communities, in our world, and in our personal lives that will be beneficial for everybody. But this will require us to think creatively, make compromises, and work together. Fortunately, this huge challenge is not insurmountable. As seen throughout history, often all it takes is one person or one small group for a transformation to occur. With just a little effort, even the smallest of change in our society can trigger a movement that inspires others to get involved. As a result, massive and extraordinary possibilities are likely for the present and for generations to come. We just need enough people who care and are committed to overcoming the challenges that are so prominent in today's society.

HEALING OURSELVES, HEALING OUR WORLD

*Although the world is full of suffering, it is also
full of the overcoming of it.*

—Helen Keller

It is extremely important that we *not* underestimate the need to develop and maintain healthy connections with one another. After all, we have a natural desire to seek belonging with others. According to the National Institute on Aging, social isolation and loneliness can lead to an increased risk of heart disease.[5] Loneliness is also often associated with cognitive decline, depression, anxiety, and suicide. I find it extremely unfortunate that we live in a world populated with millions of people, yet so many of us feel like we're all alone. More and more I hear people express that they don't have friends they can depend on.

For large portions of my life, I've also felt alone and lonely, like there was a void in my life due to the lack of connection to others. Regardless of our age, social status, race, religious affiliation, or gender, we need relationships and friendships where we feel both liked and loved. This is why we each should strive to do a better job of reaching out to people (even if it's a complete stranger) and checking on them. Sometimes just asking "How are you doing?" can mean so much to someone. Who knows, it's possible that person hasn't been sincerely asked that question in a very long time.

This leads me to another likely step to improving our society: practicing kindness. Being kind seems like a very simple thing to do on a regular basis. We can demonstrate kindness in so many ways, and both the giver and the receiver will experience benefits.

Most of us have experienced kindness, or we've done

something kind for another. Some of the most touching true-life stories we hear about are instances in which someone does something amazing for another human being that they likely didn't have to do but were inspired to anyway. To be honest, I've often found myself tearing up as I hear one of these stories; it touches my heart and my spirit.

The following are just some of the ways in which kindness can be expressed, which can go a long way toward healing one another and our world:

- Giving our time, talent, or money to help someone
- Taking the time to understand the challenges someone else may be dealing with
- Trying as hard as possible to avoid being critical, judgmental, or verbally or physically abusive, and instead using the same energy to create positive interactions
- Showing respect for one another as a fellow human and as a spiritual being
- Expressing love for others in diverse ways. I have a feeling that when each of our lives is coming to an end, if we have any regrets, it *will not* be "I should have loved less."

Forgiveness

Despite how challenging it can be, another powerful way to show kindness is through forgiveness. None of us are perfect; therefore we will all do and say things sometimes that hurt someone and that we later regret. I respect everyone's right to determine whether they want to forgive someone, but I believe that when we forgive, we free ourselves from the burden of holding on to pain, frustration, and anger. Once we are able to let go of resentment and truly forgive, we're likely to feel freer, less stressed, and happier overall.

Holding on to anger is like wrapping your hand around the blade of a knife. You probably shouldn't be holding it that way in the first place, but because you choose to hang on and squeeze tightly (perhaps out of anger), you only end up hurting yourself and creating deeper wounds.

Harboring feelings of resentment negatively impacts us mentally, emotionally, and spiritually and creates a barrier to experiencing the inner peace many of us truly desire. Forgiving someone doesn't mean we have to forget what they said or did, nor does it mean we can't still love them or that they don't love us. I am simply suggesting that forgiveness can produce amazing and long-lasting results within ourselves and within our society.

Imagine what the world would be like if we could consistently express kindness and respect for one another (especially those with different beliefs, different backgrounds, and different skin). I realize loving one another (especially if it's someone we don't know), practicing forgiveness, and treating people with respect sounds both idealistic and difficult. I'm not saying this is easy to do, especially in today's world. However, I also believe that true healing and growth aren't always easy.

During my years as a mental health professional, I've seen so many people who are experiencing varying degrees of emotional pain and personal struggles. For some, their issues could have been more manageable, or not present at all, if they were treated better by those who were an instrumental part of their lives. I believe that if we are intentional in our desire to help one another, life will be better for everyone. We will then, I believe, be more successful, live healthier lives, have stronger connections, and be happier.

CHAPTER 10

Hopes for the Future

You cannot change that which you do not accept.

—Neale Donald Walsch

It's still hard to believe it's been twenty years since I was in my master's program and conducting my first (and free) therapy sessions. In case you're not aware, as part of the typical graduate program, there are usually a certain number of practicum hours (intern hours) you are required to complete before you graduate.

Like many of my classmates, I really wanted to do well as I studied the various diagnoses, challenges, and mental health treatment modalities. I often found myself up late at night studying or working on a paper despite being physically and mentally drained from my full-time job working with kids at Challengers Boys & Girls Club in Los Angeles. At the time, it was one of the largest Boys & Girls Clubs in the country; during the school year there was a minimum of three to four hundred in attendance, and in the summer upward of seven hundred children would be enrolled.

Completing a master's program while having a full-time job became even more challenging for me once I was required to start seeing actual clients as part of my program. This meant that, with the school's assistance, I was to find a place to start working with people while under the supervision of a licensed clinician on site, as well as the guidance of the school's instructors.

As a second-year grad student, before I started seeing clients, I would hear many of my fellow classmates talking about how anxiety-ridden they were right before they conducted their first session. Many of them questioned if they would know what to do. Would they know what to say, or even how to say what may be helpful to the person sitting before them? Sometimes hearing the stories about their initial meetings made me concerned, especially since I started seeing clients a little later than many of my classmates and wondered how overwhelmed I might end up being myself.

The first intern site I started working at provided free mental health services to the gay and lesbian population in a particular part of Los Angeles. Not being a part of this community myself made me a little leery if they would accept me. I hoped that a potential client wouldn't question my sexual orientation and or feel a heterosexual was not qualified to help them with their issue. I soon found out that this would not be a problem for either of us. If I recall correctly, my first session was with a gay man, immediately followed by a couples therapy session with two gay men. I can't remember what their issues were because this was many years ago, but what I do remember is that once each session started, not only was I not nervous, but I felt both comfortable and surprisingly confident. Now please understand that just because it felt natural for me does not mean I knew exactly what to do or say the entire time. I still had a lot to learn about how to conduct a therapy session and more importantly how to help a myriad of clients with a variety of troubling issues. Despite the initial uncertainty of what it meant to conduct a therapy session, after that first evening I knew I had discovered that being a mental health professional was not only what I was meant to do but also a vital part of my life's journey.

I share this story about my beginnings in the world of therapy because looking back, I can now see the growth that I've made as a clinician, as a man, and as a human being. During the same time, I've also witnessed growth and advancement in the world of therapy. There are now more ways to treat those struggling with mental health challenges (more advanced interventions, new theoretical approaches, technological advancements, etc.). But one of the areas of progress I'm most pleased to see is that seeking mental health treatment has increasingly become more normalized and accepted, as well as less stigmatized.

Despite the concerns that I expressed in the previous chapter for people, our communities, and the world, I still strive to remain optimistic. I believe that we all not only have the potential to be healthier in mind, body, and spirit but also have within us the ability to make the necessary changes in order to better our world and our lives.

Sometimes it's challenging for me, maybe even for you as well, to always strive to be hopeful and positive about our society. A lot of this is due to seeing myself as a realist, which for me means accepting circumstances as they play out, no matter how unfortunate or negative they may be. However, my desire to continue growing, evolving, and thinking positively forces me to maintain my faith and believe anything is possible, especially those things I may not be able to see in the moment. I choose to believe that we are all capable of positive and meaningful change, and that these changes can bring about better living, better relationships, increased healing, and *ultimately* a better world for us all. I think this way because I choose to believe that many of the dreams we all hope for will be manifested during our lifetime.

MY HOPES AS A CLINICIAN

> *We choose hope over fear. We see the future not as something out of our control, but as something we can shape for the better through concerted and collective effort. We reject fatalism or cynicism when it comes to human affairs; we choose to work for the world as it should be, as our children deserve it to be.*
>
> —Barack Obama

I hope that the shame and embarrassment of going to therapy continue to decrease, especially for men and minorities. I believe it's very likely that we will continue to become more open-minded and willing to consider mental health treatment as a way to help us address many of our personal challenges.

I have hopes that even more celebrities will continue to normalize mental health treatment as they share that they, too, need and are open to receiving help. By doing this they become role models for others who were unwilling or afraid to speak to a therapist.

I hope that we can all learn to love ourselves more and that by doing so, we can also model for our children how to do the same.

I have hope that one day all people, regardless of their

race, their economic status, their insurance (or lack thereof), or their community, will have unlimited access to mental health care.

I have hopes that in the future, men, especially those of color, will increasingly acknowledge their weaknesses and their wounds and seek out treatment to find the healing they need and deserve, enabling them to become the best versions of themselves. As men address their personal challenges, this will provide an opportunity for women to experience better relationships, have healthier interactions, and receive the benefits of being loved by healthy men.

It is my hope that we can and will find ways to build resiliency in children and improve their overall coping skills, and that we will encourage children to learn the value of pushing through, the importance of overcoming challenges, and how to deal with situations when their expectations are not met.

I have hope that we will strive to identify preventative measures to keep people mentally healthy and emotionally stable, therefore avoiding the need for treatment. Ideally, by taking this approach we'll be encouraged to incorporate regular activities that take care of our minds and emotions into our lifestyles, preventing conditions like depression and anxiety from occurring, or significantly reducing their impact.

I hope, as discussed in chapter 9, that schools will play an even larger role in helping our children get prepared mentally and emotionally for life in this world. I like the idea of teachers and school administrators being able to have daily check-ins with the entire student body in order to assess whether someone is experiencing an internal struggle. I also hope that schools will develop classes at every grade level to help students improve their self-esteem, be resilient, develop coping skills, learn conflict-resolution strategies, experience the benefits of hard work, respect others, be kind, and make good decisions (which may help prevent a troubled child from hurting others). I know someone is reading this and thinking, *Shouldn't this be what parents do?* The answer is of course yes; however, will they and can they effectively teach these valuable tools? Sometimes they do; often they don't.

My hopes for the future include us *finally* realizing we are stronger as a family, community, nation, and world when we come together and support one another. I look forward to the day when we will have learned the benefits of not just thinking about ourselves but, instead, understanding we all benefit from the well-being and happiness of others. By demonstrating more compassion and empathy, we'll assuredly make our lives better on this planet.

I have hopes that every day more and more people develop the inner strength to get out of toxic situations and relationships.

My hope is that we are all able to take responsibility for our lives and the lives of others when we have the power to bring about positive change by altering our thoughts and our actions. With this hope, we will become more aware that we are shaping our lives every second, every minute, every hour, and every day by the things we think about and the actions we repeatedly take.

As we continue going forward in our lives, taking advantage of the resources that so many of us have at our fingertips, may we use these tools without feeling weak or wondering what others think. This includes gaining help and insight from books, life coaches, therapists, podcasts, mentors, seminars, retreats—anything that helps us grow, overcome, and heal. Never before in history have we had so many different tools available to assist us. Just as we feed our bodies on a regular basis, may we also prioritize nourishing our minds and our spirits.

I hope that we will decrease our current dependency on drugs. This includes recreational drugs as well as those overprescribed for medicinal purposes. Wouldn't it be great if, in the near future, we are able to identify other, more natural ways to treat mental and physical health issues? I hope people will use more positive ways to cope with personal challenges, instead of using drugs as a way of escaping feelings or experiences.

I hope that in the future, both young and old are able to embrace the value of personal growth by being willing to step out of their comfort zones—by being willing to try new things in order to improve their self-confidence, experience a higher quality of life, and achieve goals they may have once thought impossible.

I have hopes that we will stop rushing to judge the actions or words of others, especially when we know nothing about them or their situations. Instead, may we seek to understand before we criticize, may we choose to hug instead of hit, to love instead of hate.

It's my hope that we will finally stop judging ourselves so harshly or being overly concerned about how we are viewed by others.

And finally, I have hopes that starting now and going forward into the future, we will spend far more time and energy living in love instead of fear.

Of course, these are not *all* of my hopes for the future, but I believe incorporating some of these ideas is not a bad place to start. In the meantime, I'll continue wishing, hoping, and praying for the best for us all.

FINAL THOUGHTS

*Growth comes from focus on our own lessons,
not on someone else's.*

—Marianne Williamson

In more ways than you know, writing a book about what I've learned being a mental health therapist has been one of the most daunting things I've ever attempted. However, I pushed through for several years, often getting up at 5:00 a.m. because I truly felt I was being guided to do so. In going forward with this book, I had to reflect and dig deep to find ways to really capture the many lessons that I've learned, working with a variety of people with unique personalities, varied life experiences, and challenging personal situations. One does not have to be a mental health professional to know how many things can be learned from the myriad of people in our lives.

The late Wayne Dyer, a self-help author and speaker, often said, "When the student is ready, the teacher will appear."[1] I believe there are many times in which we find ourselves at a certain point in our lives when the right person or people will show up to help us, providing the insight or guidance we need. I believe "the teacher" comes in many forms, which may be another person, but they also may show up in the form of a book, film, song, poem, podcast, billboard, or post on social media. As I've gotten older, I've come to understand that our teachers are all around us and can also come in the form of a personal experience or challenge.

While serving as a therapist for two decades, I have been delighted to discover how much my clients, friends, family, and even coworkers have either been amazing teachers or simply contributed to my personal growth. When we work to help others, it's hard not to simultaneously benefit from the experience in ways seen or unseen, known or unknown. As we experience each day, we continue to discover what we want in our lives and what we don't want. We hopefully come to realize the person we want to become or the person we want to avoid becoming. We learn from the people who emotionally feed us as well as the people who drain us. We learn about situations that are toxic and harmful and those that are uplifting and empowering. Hopefully, from all that we are experiencing, we gain insights to help us lead better lives.

LET'S ALL EXPERIENCE PERSONAL GROWTH

I'm convinced that many things we go through provide opportunities for awareness, insight, and personal growth, leading to positive change for ourselves or for those around us.

Many recent events have made us question who we are as people and as a society—situations where some of us have questioned the direction of humanity. Common sense sometimes doesn't appear to be as common as we once thought it was. I see wonderful displays of empathy and compassion everywhere while simultaneously experiencing what, in my opinion, appears to be an increasing amount of ignorance, selfishness, greed, and an unwillingness to understand or forgive. It seems we don't value or understand the fact that love surrounds us, connects us, and is available at any given moment for us to experience, give, or receive.

I've heard it said that how an individual deals with circumstances says a lot about who they are as a person. Likewise, circumstances and how we deal with them can also reveal who we are as a society. If we are able to grow as individuals, we will have a greater ability to work together and solve many of the problems we continue to struggle with in our world.

We Can All Use Some Healing

To varying degrees, we all have wounds that need healing. We have all experienced heartbreak, disappointment, fear, struggle, pain (emotionally and physically), doubt, lack, and loss. Since we share so many of these experiences, I can't help but believe that they are a part of life and what we are supposed to *grow through*.

Perhaps this gamut of situations we're often forced to deal with is just a part of all of our life's journey. Perhaps there are situations where healing requires us to learn how to push through and overcome challenges, ultimately moving toward our highest potential. Maybe part of healing and growing is learning to accept certain aspects of life and not be so quick to push back or resist. Perhaps healing would be a more likely outcome if we invested as much time and energy into nurturing our soul and serving others as we do pursuing worldly desires and thinking about ourselves. What if, instead of spending so much time doing things that do not serve our highest good, such as spending hours on social media or watching television, we spent half as much time engaging in prayer or meditation, or reading books that promote mental, emotional, and spiritual healing?

I Am Grateful

Despite the challenges of trying to help people as a mental health professional, I am truly grateful to have a job where I can make a positive difference in the lives of others. This may be tough to imagine, but when I help others grow, heal, and overcome their challenges, I'm also learning how to do the same for myself. Since becoming a marriage and family therapist, I have significantly increased my ability to display compassion and concern for others. I've become better—not perfect—at not judging others and have evolved into a better listener as I hear my client's stories, empathize with them, and respect their journeys.

It has been a gift for me to serve as my clients' therapist. I only hope and pray that I've been able to provide them with whatever they were in most need of. There is tremendous value that we all gain when we serve others or something bigger than ourselves, especially when the ultimate goal of the service is rooted in expressions of love, unity, and kindness.

There are so many broken, suffering, and hurt people in this world. Sometimes I wish I could simply take a giant blanket of comfort and use it to cover the entire planet. Unfortunately, I can't do that, but instead I'm going to continue doing what I can (and hopefully you will too). I will continue dedicating my life to trying to be the best mental health clinician possible. I will continue striving to be a person who expresses empathy and compassion. I will continue striving to be the best husband, friend, brother, teacher, and human being that I am able to be.

In the meantime, I will encourage others to strive to be

the best version of themselves as well. I hope that I have said something in these pages that has provided even a small bit of encouragement, hope, new insight, and a desire for continued healing and growth. A big part of growth is being willing to learn about others and, more importantly, being willing to learn about oneself.

Let's Remember . . .

I hope we all remember life is fragile, precious, and finite. Even the smallest of moments can be special and amazing. There are only a certain number of sunsets remaining that we each will experience. There are a definitive number of hugs, kisses, and other wonderful moments that we have left before we transition to whatever the next phase of living is. It's important to appreciate each and every day that we have on this current plane of existence. Today is the only day we truly have, so why not do the best we possibly can to enjoy it and express love to others?

No matter what a client may be experiencing, no matter what you or I may be experiencing, no matter what the perceived challenges may be, there is still beauty in the world. To truly see the wonders that surround us, all we need to do is be willing to open our hearts and eyes and take a good look around. This beauty may be in the form of a child's smile as they play in the park, or in the sound of a hearty laugh. The beauty can be witnessed in the setting of the sun, a hug from a loved one, or a night full of stars. We are always surrounded by things we're taking for granted and should probably appreciate more.

There is a lot more that could be said about the topics that I've discussed in this book. I strongly encourage anyone interested in learning more to take advantage of the many people, books, and resources that are available to us. If you're looking for a starting point, two books that I think are life changing and thought provoking are *Life Lessons: Two Experts on Death and Dying Teach Us About the Mysteries of Life and Living* by Elisabeth Kübler-Ross and David Kessler, and *The Rabbit Effect: Live Longer, Happier, and Healthier with the Groundbreaking Science of Kindness* by Kelli Harding.

I plan to continue striving to help others, and I hope that in doing so, I continue to grow and evolve as well. A large part of my life's purpose is to strive to do three things: increase our understanding of one another, promote unity (regardless of our differences), and assist in any way I can with healing the mental and emotional wounds of others. I hope I have been able to do some of those things by writing this book. Equally important, I hope that you are willing to join me, in some large or small way, to do the same.

May everyone's life be filled with peace, love, healing and growing.

ACKNOWLEDGMENTS

I would first like to give thanks to what I believe is the divine intelligence that makes our lives and existence possible. It is also the same presence that connects us to one another, allows us to know and experience love, and whom I frequently refer to as Comforter, Creator, Source, and God. I believe it is Spirit that both nudged me into creating this book and provided me with the words that I hope can touch others in ways that promote insight, growth, and healing.

I feel like I cannot go any further without next mentioning and thanking my angel on earth: my beautiful, intelligent, funny, kind, and loving wife, Laurie. You are without a doubt my best friend. So much of who I am today and the abundance of blessings in my life are because of you. I don't believe there is any way that I would be where I am now, personally or professionally, without you being by my side. "Thank you" does not express how truly appreciative and fortunate I am to have shared my life's journey with you. Please know that my heart is, and will always be, filled with gratitude and love for you.

To my mother, who, despite the limited income she made working in small diners when we were young, was able to take care of my sister and me and provide everything we needed. And although she was unable to obtain an education beyond the seventh grade, she still produced two children who both went on to get their master's degrees and have wonderful careers positively impacting others.

Thank you, Rose, for being my big sister and helping me in so many ways when we were young, including with my schoolwork. But a much bigger thanks is necessary for the incredible sacrifices you (along with your husband, Mr. Marshall) have made by taking care of our mother when she began experiencing dementia and various other debilitating conditions. I may not say it as much as I should, but hopefully you know I love you.

Gary and Elliot, not only have you guys been wonderful nephews, but I've watched you both become good men and present fathers to my great-nieces and great-nephews. I truly appreciate how our relationships have grown over the years, allowing us to be amazing friends as well as family. I would also like to mention people who've been a part of your lives, past and present: Kimberly (Elliot's wife), Jadon, and their families.

Thank you to my surrogate family. We may not be related by blood, but that does not change the incredible amount of love we've shared and have for one another. Thank you for adding so much value and meaning to my life: Auntie Joyce; Uncle Walter; my "nieces," Kori and Marissa ("Angie"); and my "Lil Sis," Kandi (along with her kids, my nephew and niece Kendall and Koko).

When I think about the many friends who've added so much value to my life, I have to begin with "The Crew." This unique, fun, intelligent, and supportive group consists of Kathy Kidd, Jason, Wilton Jr., Ramon, Valerie Battiest-Danzy, and Traci Stanford. Although there are many reasons why it's been nearly impossible for us to all be together like the "old days," we've always been there for one another and have had some amazing times to reflect on during our thirty-plus years of friendship.

Katrina Wright, you have truly been one of my closest and best friends. Throughout the many years, no matter where either of us lived in the US, we always made time to check in with one another, often sharing our dating struggles and the unique, bizarre, or entertaining people we found ourselves going out with.

Other friends whom I must mention that I have always considered special and an important part of my past, especially during my college years. This includes Tonya, who became a part of my life during our days at Southern Illinois University in Carbondale; Eric, Pam, and the entire Cunningham family, including Moni (your transition happened way too soon), Octavia, and Emerson (continue resting in peace). You guys always made me feel welcomed, cared for, and a part of your family. Jackie Wittenberg, who would've guessed we'd still be friends after all these years? And Robert "Uncle Rob" Carter, my former hapkido partner, also known as "Robbie C."

Jeanne Sparrow, our friendship began many years ago while working at WGCI radio. I've always been an admirer of your intellect, your caring heart, and your many talents. But what I appreciate most is that despite us talking sporadically and only seeing one another once a year, our connection has remained strong and based in love.

To those who became my friends while I was living in Southern California and whom I remain close to today (even if we don't get to talk to each other often). This group of wonderful people includes Elyce Strong Mann, Elena McGill, Lorie Overstreet Squire, Christina Mathis, Matt, Carmen Jones Madison, and Sheree Thompkins. Thank you for being a part of my life and filling the void of loneliness that I so often experienced before we met.

Thanks to Ancestry.com, I found and formed relationships with relatives, including my niece Yolanda M. Peters (let's get together soon, please) and a significant number of family members who reside in the UK that I had no idea existed. Carol, my UK cousin who lives in New York, it's been great spending the past few years getting to know you and your family. And to my other "cousins" overseas (Marie Roy, Michelle Brown, Anthony, Christine, Nessa, and Melanie South), I look forward to when I'll finally meet you guys in person instead of chatting through Facebook, emails, WhatsApp, or video calls.

I would definitely be remiss if I did not mention my wife Laurie's family, who, from the moment we met, welcomed me with open arms and love. This starts with her parents, William and Juanita; her sister Angela; her nephew Brandon; cousin Evelyn (continue resting in peace), and other extended family members, including Dorothy, Carolyn, Tony, Tanya, Sonny, Sharon, AJ, Christopher ("Chris"), Takiya, Ronnie, Theo, and Ebony.

Since relocating to Georgia, I've been blessed to develop some really great friendships with some really great people. This includes my wife's best friend, Kishya (along with her family); Kimberly; her mother, Beverly Hill Shelley; Alicia Butler Pierre; and Will and Nicole Hill. You guys started out as friends and have now become a part of my Atlanta family.

I'd like to thank Regina Zabel for not only being a friend but also allowing me to be a part of the team that is Renewed Journey Counseling Services (for more than ten years), where I've had the opportunity to work with some awesome individuals who truly care about doing a good job for their clients. Being there has enabled me to continue learning and growing as a mental health professional.

Patricia Harwell and Trudy Post Sprunk, you both were wonderful supervisors who helped me during the earlier part of my career, contributing to me becoming the therapist I am today.

To those who have been my clients (as well as those whom I have mentored), thank you for trusting me enough to share so much of your personal lives and struggles. You opened your minds and your hearts to us working together in order to achieve your goals and, more importantly, to heal and to grow. You welcomed my support and agreed to meet the challenges that I presented to assist you with moving forward. And finally, thank you for unknowingly providing opportunities for me to continue learning how to be a better listener, husband, clinician, and man.

Special thanks to Darnah Mercieca, Kathleen McIntosh, Rachael Brandenburg, Rikki Jump, and Mark Chait for working with me during the first half of this project that would go on to become this book. I must also mention Jenna Love Schrader who was also a great help.

I am also extremely grateful for my amazing team at Girl Friday Productions, which included Karen McNally, Sara Spees Addicott, Abi Pollokoff, Georgie Hockett, Sarah Breeding, Karen Parkin, and a host of others who I haven't met who all worked together to help me complete my story by making this book a reality and dream come true.

And finally, I know you can't read this (it would be cool if you could), but I have to mention my English golden retriever, Buddy! You are truly my best pal, my road dog, and my wrestling buddy. Thanks for the many hours you would lie right by my side (as you're doing as I write this) while I worked tirelessly trying to share my thoughts and experiences that would eventually become this book.

If I missed anyone, please accept my apologies and know that it was likely due to my poor memory and has absolutely nothing to do with the role that you have played in my life.

NOTES

Chapter 2: Lessons Learned About Anxiety and Depression

1. "The Serenity Prayer and Twelve Step Recovery: Finding the Balance between Acceptance and Change", Hazelden Betty Ford Foundation, October 11, 2018, https://www.hazeldenbettyford .org/articles/the-serenity-prayer.
2. "Hopeful Thinking: Comparison Is the Thief of Joy," *The Sun*, October 22, 2022, https://www.lowellsun.com/2022/10/22 /hopeful-thinking-comparison-is-the-thief-of-joy/.

Chapter 3: Lessons Learned About Couples Therapy

1. Gary Chapman, *The 5 Love Languages*, accessed September 4, 2022, https://5lovelanguages.com/.
2. *The Oprah Winfrey Show*, Season 9, Episode 1, uploaded by OWN Network June 4, 2023, https://www.youtube.com /watch?v=E2uDWu_OEus.
3. "Infidelity," American Association for Marriage and Family Therapy, accessed September 4, 2022, https://www.aamft.org /consumer_updates/infidelity.aspx.

Chapter 4: Lessons Learned About Nonromantic Relationships

1. Michael Leonard, "Robin Williams Quotes That Will Help You Find Meaning in Your Life," *Fearless Soul*, July 23, 2018, https://iamfearlesssoul.com/robin-williams-quotes/.
2. "Social Isolation, Loneliness in Older People Pose Health Risks," National Institute on Aging, April 23, 2019, https://www.nia.nih.gov/news/social-isolation-loneliness-older-people-pose-health-risks.
3. Vivek Murthy, "Work and the Loneliness Epidemic," *Harvard Business Review* (2017): 3–7.
4. "The Only Way to Have a Friend Is to Be One," BrainyQuote, accessed September 4, 2021, https://www.brainyquote.com/quotes/ralph_waldo_emerson_100740.
5. Joel Manby, *Love Works: Seven Timeless Principles for Effective Leaders* (Grand Rapids, MI: Zondervan, 2012).

Chapter 5: Lessons Learned About Men and Therapy

1. *Spider-Man*, directed by Sam Raimi (Columbia Pictures, Marvel Enterprises, and Laura Ziskin Productions, 2002).
2. E. P. Terlizzi and T. Norris, *Mental Health Treatment among Adults, United States, 2020*, NCHS Data Brief no. 419 (Hyattsville, MD: National Center for Health Statistics, 2021).

Chapter 6: Lessons Learned About Children and Adolescents

1. David G. Myers and C. Nathan DeWall, "Developing through the Life Span," *Psychology in Everyday Life*, 6th ed. (New York: Worth Publishers, 2023), 85.
2. Ibid., 85.

Chapter 8: Challenges in Treatment

1. "42 Worrying Workplace Stress Statistics," The American

Institute of Stress, September 25, 2019, https://www.stress
.org/42-worrying-workplace-stress-statistics#:~:text=83%25
%20of%20US%20workers%20suffer,about%20their%20
work%2Dlife%20balance.

Chapter 9: Concerns for Our Communities and World

1. "Fact Sheet: President Biden to Announce Strategy to Address
   Our National Mental Health Crisis, As Part of Unity Agenda
   in his First State of the Union," The White House, March 1,
   2022, https://www.whitehouse.gov/briefing-room/statements
   -releases/2022/03/01/fact-sheet-president-biden-to-announce
   -strategy-to-address-our-national-mental-health-crisis-as-part
   -of-unity-agenda-in-his-first-state-of-the-union/.
2. "The Doctor Is Out," National Alliance on Mental Illness,
   accessed September 23, 2022, https://www.nami.org/Support
   -Education/Publications-Reports/Public-Policy-Reports/The
   -Doctor-is-Out/DoctorIsOut.
3. R. C. Kessler, P. Berglund, O. Demler, et al., "Life-Time Prevalence
   and Age-of-Onset Distribution of DSM-IV Disorders in the
   National Co-morbidity Survey Replication," *Archives of General
   Psychiatry* 62 (2005): 593–602.
4. Pat Croskerry, "To Err Is Human—and Let's Not Forget It,"
   Canadian Medical Association Journal, 182, no. 5 (2010): 524.
   https://doi.org/10.1503/cmaj.100270.
5. "Social Isolation, Loneliness in Older People Pose Health Risks,"
   National Institute on Aging, April 23, 2019, https://www.nia
   .nih.gov/news/social-isolation-loneliness-older-people-pose
   -health-risks.

Final Thoughts

1. Wayne Dyer, *Wishes Fulfilled: Mastering the Art of Manifesting*
   (New York: Hay House, Inc., 2012), chap. 3, Kindle.

ABOUT THE AUTHOR

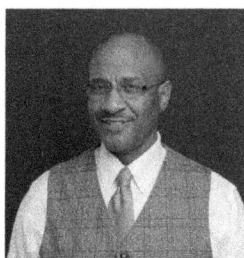

F. Francis Jones is a licensed marriage and family therapist in the state of Georgia who has helped clients overcome a variety of personal issues, diagnoses, and challenges for more than twenty years. He has provided therapy services to individual children, adolescents, and adults, as well as families and couples, while striving to help them navigate a path toward healing and becoming the best possible versions of themselves. Prior to becoming a clinician, Jones worked in radio and television for fourteen years, during which time he gained valuable experience interacting with people from all walks of life. He currently works in private practice and also teaches psychology as an adjunct instructor at a community college. His life's mission has always been to make a positive difference in the lives of others in the hope of making the world a better place for all.

To learn more, visit www.ffrancisjones.com.